Hereditary Colorectal Cancer

Guest Editor

STEVEN GALLINGER, MD, MSc, FRCS(C)

SURGICAL ONCOLOGY CLINICS OF NORTH AMERICA

www.surgonc.theclinics.com

Consulting Editor
NICHOLAS J. PETRELLI, MD

October 2009 • Volume 18 • Number 4

SAUNDERS an imprint of ELSEVIER, Inc.

W.B. SAUNDERS COMPANY

A Division of Elsevier Inc.

1600 John F. Kennedy Boulevard ● Suite 1800 ● Philadelphia, PA 19103-2899

http://www.theclinics.com

SURGICAL ONCOLOGY CLINICS OF NORTH AMERICA Volume 18, Number 4

October 2009 ISSN 1055-3207, ISBN-13: 978-1-4377-1390-9, ISBN-10: 1-4377-1390-4

Editor: Catherine Bewick
Developmental Editor: Theresa Collier

Surgical Oncology Clinics of North America (ISSN 1055-3207) is published quarterly by Elsevier Inc., 360 Park Avenue South, New York, NY 10010-1710. Months of publication are January, April, July, and October. Subscription prices are $218.00 per year (US individuals), $333.00 (US institutions) $110.00 (US student/resident), $251.00 (Canadian individuals), $414.00 (Canadian institutions), $158.00 (Canadian student/resident), $314.00 (foreign individuals), $414.00 (foreign institutions), and $158.00 (foreign student/resident). Foreign air speed delivery is included in all *Clinics* subscription prices. All prices are subject to change without notice. POSTMASTER: Send address changes to *Surgical Oncology Clinics of North America*, Elsevier Health Sciences Division, Subscription Customer Service, 3251 Riverport Lane, Maryland Heights, MO 63043. **Customer Service: 1-800-654-2452 (U.S. and Canada); 314-447-8871 (outside U.S. and Canada). Fax: 314-447-8029. E-mail: journalscustomerservice-usa@elsevier.com (for print support); journalsonlinesupport-usa@elsevier.com (for online support).**

Reprints. For copies of 100 or more, of articles in this publication, please contact the Commercial Reprints Department, Elsevier Inc., 360 Park Avenue South, New York, New York 10010-1710. Tel. 212-633-3813; Fax: 212-462-1935; E-mail: reprints@elsevier.com.

Surgical Oncology Clinics of North America is covered in *MEDLINE/PubMed (Index Medicus)* and *EMBASE/Excerpta Medica, Current Contents/Clinical Medicine,* and *ISI/BIOMED.*

Printed and bound by CPI Group (UK) Ltd, Croydon, CR0 4YY

Transferred to Digital Print 2012

Contributors

CONSULTING EDITOR

NICHOLAS J. PETRELLI, MD
Bank of America Endowed Medical Director, Helen F. Graham Cancer Center at Christiana Care Health System, Newark, Delaware; Professor of Surgery, Thomas Jefferson University, Philadelphia, Pennsylvania

GUEST EDITOR

STEVEN GALLINGER, MD, MSc, FRCS(C)
Senior Scientist, Samuel Lunenfeld Research Institute, Mount Sinai Hospital; Professor of Surgery and Head of Hepatobiliary/Pancreatic Surgical Oncology, University Health Network, Toronto, Ontario, Canada

AUTHORS

CHRISTOPHER AMOS, PhD, FACMG
Head, Section of Computational and Genetic Epidemiology, and Informatics, Department of Epidemiology; Annie Laurie Howard Professor of Epidemiology, Bioinformatics and Computational Biology; University of Texas, MD Anderson Cancer Center, Houston, Texas

MELYSSA ARONSON, MS, CCGC, CGC
Senior Genetic Counselor, Mount Sinai Hospital; Dr. Zane Cohen Digestive Disease Clinical Research Centre; Familial Gastrointestinal Cancer Registry; Instructor, Department of Medical Genetics and Microbiology, University of Toronto, Toronto, Ontario, Canada

JAMES CHURCH, MB, ChB, FRACS
Director, Sanford R. Weiss Center for Hereditary Colorectal Neoplasia, Digestive Diseases Institute, Cleveland Clinic Foundation, Cleveland, Ohio

MALCOLM G. DUNLOP, MD
Professor, Colon Cancer Genetics Group, Institute of Genetics and Molecular Medicine, University of Edinburgh and MRC Human Genetics Unit, Western General Hospital, Edinburgh, United Kingdom

SUSAN M. FARRINGTON, PhD
Colon Cancer Genetics Group, Institute of Genetics and Molecular Medicine, University of Edinburgh and MRC Human Genetics Unit, Western General Hospital, Edinburgh, United Kingdom

ROBERT GRYFE, MD, PhD, FRSCSC
Assistant Professor, Department of Surgery, Mount Sinai Hospital and The Samuel Lunenfeld Research Institute, University of Toronto, Toronto, Ontario, Canada

HEATHER HAMPEL, MS, CGC
Clinical Associate Professor and Associate Clinical Director, Department of Internal Medicine, Division of Human Genetics, The Ohio State University Comprehensive Cancer Center, Columbus, Ohio

MARK A. JENKINS, PhD
Associate Professor, Centre for MEGA Epidemiology School of Population Health, The University of Melbourne, Australia

LOÏC LE MARCHAND, MD, PhD
Professor of Epidemiology Program, Cancer Research Center of Hawaii, University of Hawaii, Honolulu, Hawaii

NORALANE M. LINDOR, MD
Professor of Medical Genetics and Consultant, Department of Medical Genetics, Mayo Clinic, Rochester, Minnesota

PATRICK M. LYNCH, JD, MD
Professor of Medicine, Department of Gastrointestinal Medicine, Hepatology and Nutrition, University of Texas MD Anderson Cancer Center, Houston, Texas

THOMAS J. McGARRITY, MD
Chief, Division of Gastroenterology and Hepatology; Professor of Medicine, Department of Medicine, Penn State Hershey Medical Center, Hershey, Pennsylvania

MIGUEL A. RODRIGUEZ-BIGAS, MD, FACS
Professor of Surgery, Department of Surgical Oncology, University of Texas MD Anderson Cancer Center, Houston, Texas

KERRINGTON D. SMITH, MD
Assistant Professor of Surgery, Division of Surgical Oncology, Dartmouth-Hitchcock Medical Center, Lebanon, New Hampshire

Contents

> Cancer is a genetic disease in which the clonal accumulation of genetic alterations confers a cell with the malignant characteristics of uncontrolled growth, local invasiveness, and metastastic potential. Studies of colorectal cancer and its precursor lesion, the adenomatous polyp, have served as the cornerstone in advancing knowledge of cancer molecular genetics. The past 30 years have ushered in an era of revolutionary increases in understanding colorectal cancer genetics. In the future, it is hoped that the tremendous recent gains made in understanding colorectal cancer genetics will allow for significant, tailored chemoprevention and treatment of this common malignancy.

> Patients with FAP are guaranteed to have one major abdominal surgery in their life. They are also subject to cancers and benign disorders in other organ systems, some of which can be life threatening. Steering a course through life while avoiding preventable disease and complications of treatment, and maintaining good quality of life is a challenge for health care givers, patients, and their families. A successful voyage calls for clinical cooperation between providers and patients, education and understanding, and expertise and experience. FAP patients and families should be involved in a registry or genetic center, not to the exclusion of local practitioners but to their benefit. In this way the best of care is given and the best of outcomes ensured.

> This article reviews the role of defective base excision repair, and MUTYH specifically, in colorectal cancer etiology and discusses the consequences of MUTYH gene defects, with particular emphasis on clinical relevance to

A variety of syndromes confer increased risk for intestinal polyp development, outside the more commonly occurring syndromes. Each of these uncommon syndromes predispose to pathognomonic histologies that are uncommonly observed. Accurate diagnosis of these syndromes is contingent on higher-level pathology review, evaluation of signs and symptoms beyond sole consideration of the polyps, and collection of a detailed family history. When a genetic mutation can be identified in the proband, the management of intestinal and extra-intestinal cancer screening can be more appropriately tailored.

Genome-wide association studies (GWAS) provide a powerful new approach to identify common, low-penetrance susceptibility loci without prior knowledge of biologic function. Results from three GWAS conducted in populations of European ancestry are available for colorectal cancer (CRC). These studies have identified 11 disease loci that, for the majority, were not previously suspected to be related to CRC. The proportions of the familial and population risks explained by these loci are small and they currently are not useful for risk prediction. However, the power of these studies was low, indicating that a number of other loci may be identified in new ongoing GWAS, and in pooled analyses. Thus, the risk prediction ability of susceptibility markers identified in GWAS for CRC may improve as more variants are discovered. This may, in turn, have important implications for targeting high-risk individuals for colonoscopy screening.

The impression that genetic testing for an inherited colorectal cancer syndrome involves a simple blood test masks the complex issues that surround this type of testing. This article explores the ethical, legal, and psychosocial implications of genetic testing and the role of genetic counseling through the genetic testing process.

This article focuses on genetic testing for hereditary colorectal cancer syndromes. Genetic testing is now available in North America for all of the known hereditary colorectal cancer genes. In addition, most of these tests have improved significantly in the past few years with the inclusion of techniques to detect large rearrangements. As a result, clinicians are in a better position than ever to help families with these syndromes to identify the underlying genetic cause. This identification will ensure that they receive appropriate management, and will enable their relatives to determine their precise risks and to tailor their cancer surveillance.

Kerrington D. Smith and Miguel A. Rodriguez-Bigas

Surgery remains the mainstay of treatment for patients who develop colorectal cancer (CRC) in the setting of a hereditary CRC syndrome. In patients with a hereditary CRC syndrome, surgery can be prophylactic, therapeutic with curative intent, and, in some cases, palliative. The type and extent of surgical resection in familial adenomatous polyposis (FAP) and in the Lynch syndrome is influenced by differences in the natural history of carcinogenesis between the two syndromes and by the effectiveness of and patient compliance with available surveillance strategies. In this article, the surgical options for the management of patients with FAP and Lynch syndrome are discussed.

RELATED INTEREST

Surgical Clinics of North America, February 2009 (Vol. 89, Number 1)
Multidisciplinary Approach to Cancer Care
K.M. Brown and M. Shoup, *Guest Editors*

THE CLINICS ARE NOW AVAILABLE ONLINE!

Access your subscription at:
www.theclinics.com

Foreword

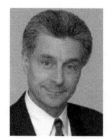

Nicholas J. Petrelli, MD
Consulting Editor

This issue of the *Surgical Oncology Clinics of North America* is dedicated to hereditary colorectal cancer. The guest editor is Steven Gallinger, MD, who is professor of surgery at the University of Toronto.

In 2009, an estimated 106,100 new cases of colon cancer and approximately 40,870 cases of rectal cancer will occur, and 49,920 people will die from colon and rectal cancer. Despite these statistics, mortality from colon cancer has decreased slightly over the past 30 years, possibly because of earlier diagnosis through screening and better treatment modalities. In the general population, the lifetime risk of colorectal cancer is approximately 5% to 6%. Patients who have two or more first- or second-degree relatives with colorectal cancer make up approximately 20% of all patients with this disease. Approximately 5% to 10% of the total annual colorectal cancer cases are inherited in an autosomal dominant manner, however. There is no question that the most important issue leading to the diagnosis of hereditary colorectal cancer is a thorough family history. Individual knowledge of family history is probably the most important factor for health today. Hereditary colorectal cancer can be separated into two global categories based on the location of the cancer. Colorectal cancers involving the distal large intestine are more likely to harbor mutations in the adenomatous polyposis coli, p53, and K-ras genes and in general behave more aggressively. Alternatively, proximal colorectal cancers are more likely to possess microsatellite instability, have mutations in the mismatched repair genes, and behave in a less aggressive manner, as in hereditary nonpolyposis colorectal cancer. Familial adenomatous polyposis and the majority of sporadic cases can be considered a paradigm for the distal class of colorectal cancers whereas hereditary nonpolyposis colorectal cancer can represent the proximal class or category of cancers.

Dr. Gallinger has put together an outstanding group of authors in this issue of the *Surgical Oncology Clinics of North America*. The article by Smith and Rodriguez-Bigas, entitled, "The Role of Surgery in Familial Adenomatous Polyposis and Hereditary Nonpolyposis Colorectal Cancer," is an excellent discussion of these two entities. Drs. Smith and Rodriguez-Bigas are from the Department of Surgical Oncology at

Surg Oncol Clin N Am 18 (2009) xi–xii
doi:10.1016/j.soc.2009.09.002   **surgonc.theclinics.com**

the MD Anderson Cancer Center. An article by Noralane Lindor, MD, from the Department of Medical Genetics at the Mayo Clinic, entitled, "Familial Colorectal Cancer Type X," also presents an outstanding discussion.

I am sure readers will also enjoy the other articles in this edition of *Surgical Oncology Clinics of North America*. As I have stated in my previous forewords, this edition is an outstanding one for individuals in training in all fields of medicine.

Nicholas J. Petrelli, MD
Helen F. Graham Cancer Center
4701 Ogletown-Stanton Road
Suite 1213
Newark, DE 19713, USA

Department of Surgery
Jefferson Medical College
1021 Walnut Street
Philadelphia, PA 19107, USA

E-mail address:
npetrelli@christianacare.org (N.J. Petrelli)

Preface

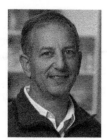

Steven Gallinger, MD, MSc, FRCS(C)
Guest Editor

Brute force genetic linkage efforts, combined with scientific and technological advances in deciphering the human genome during the 1990s, are now beginning to bear fruit in the clinic. This is evident in the current decade as we appreciate the clinical translatability of discoveries relevant to identifying and managing subjects with hereditary colorectal cancer. This issue of *Surgical Oncology Clinics of North America* provides a practical update on this subject and a glimpse of further advances in the field.

The identification of mutations of the *APC* and mismatch repair genes as the causes of familial adenomatous polyposis and hereditary nonpolyposis colorectal cancer, respectively, has made a significant impact on genetic counseling, cancer surveillance, and tailored surgical approaches for gene carriers and their relatives. More recently, MYH-associated polyposis has also been characterized as a cause of high-penetrant colorectal neoplasia with a unique pattern of recessive inheritance.

The aforementioned genetic conditions and other rare syndromes described herein explain only 2% to 3% of all colorectal cancer and only a small fraction of hereditary cases. What syndrome or syndromes are associated with the remainder? Are there additional undiscovered high-penetrant genes? How do environmental factors interact with genetic variation? These questions remain for future generations of scientists to answer. In the meantime, the term *familial colorectal cancer type X* has been coined to describe a likely heterogeneous group of families with higher risk for colorectal cancer, but not associated with tumor microsatellite instability.

If we assume that almost all cases of cancer have a genetic component, then even sporadic cases of colorectal cancer should be explained by germline genomic variation. The era of genome-wide association studies is upon us and first-generation interrogation of the human genome has revealed curious findings that are enlightening our understanding of the contribution of common alleles to colorectal cancer risk. As more dense single nucleotide polymorphism chips and other tools for exploring epigenetic variation are developed and employed, it is certain that novel genetic models of risk

Surg Oncol Clin N Am 18 (2009) xiii–xiv
doi:10.1016/j.soc.2009.09.001
1055-3207/09/$ – see front matter © 2009 Elsevier Inc. All rights reserved.

will be created for individualized assessment of colorectal cancer risk. Moreover, the role of genetic counselors will be expanded as the scientific and medical community translates these findings for the public.

Steven Gallinger, MD, MSc, FRCS(C)
Samuel Lunenfeld Research Institute
Toronto General Hospital
Suite 206-10 Eaton North
200 Elisabeth Street
Toronto, M5G2C4
Ontario, Canada

E-mail address:
Steven.gallinger@uhn.on.ca (S. Gallinger)

Overview of Colorectal Cancer Genetics

Robert Gryfe, MD, PhD, FRSCSC

KEYWORDS

- Colorectal cancer genetics • Tumor suppressor genes
- Oncogenes • Chromosomal instability
- Microsatellite instability • CpG island methylation

In the United States, colorectal cancer remains the third most commonly diagnosed cancer, accounting for 10% of newly diagnosed malignancies.[1] Similarly, colorectal cancer is the second leading cause of cancer deaths in the United States and accounts for 9% of annual cancer deaths in both genders.

Cancer is now known to be a genetic disease in which the clonal accumulation of genetic alterations allows uncontrolled growth, evasion of cell death, local invasiveness, and metastatic potential.[2–5] The genetics of cancer usually refers to the somatic genetic alterations that occur in normal adult cells leading to malignancy but may also include inherited germline genetic alterations in the case of familial cancer syndromes. No cancer better exemplifies current knowledge of the molecular genetic basis of neoplasia than does cancer of colon and rectum.

HISTORICAL PERSPECTIVE

Although the past 30 years have witnessed a revolution in the understanding of cancer genetics, the notion that chromosomal abnormalities may cause normal cells to become cancerous dates back to the late nineteenth and early twentieth century work of David Paul von Hansemann and Theodor Boveri.[6] In 1890, Hansemann coined the term, *anaplasia*, in describing the asymmetric nuclear divisions that he observed in human epithelial cancers. He further observed that the asymmetric mitoses present in cancer cells were accompanied by increased cell growth potential and loss of cell differentiation. Although often credited with the chromosomal theory of tumors, Boveri (who previously had established the identity of the chromosomes and harmonized Mendel's laws by describing how, through fertilization, haploid gametes produce the diploid chromosomal status) explicitly cited and popularized Hansemann's work in his 1914 book, *Origin of Malignant Tumors*.

The same era that produced the first descriptions of chromosomal abnormalities accompanying neoplasia also brought forward the first published descriptions of

Department of Surgery, Mount Sinai Hospital and The Samuel Lunenfeld Research Institute, University of Toronto, 600 University Avenue, Suite 455, Toronto, Ontario, Canada M5G 1X5
E-mail address: rgryfe@mtsinai.on.ca

Surg Oncol Clin N Am 18 (2009) 573–583
doi:10.1016/j.soc.2009.08.004
1055-3207/09/$ – see front matter © 2009 Elsevier Inc. All rights reserved.

surgonc.theclinics.com

the inherited colorectal cancer syndromes that would later become known as familial adenomatous polyposis (FAP) and hereditary nonpolyposis colorectal cancer (HNPCC). In terms of FAP, in 1892, Harrison Cripps, a British surgeon, reported on "disseminated polypus of the rectum" in 17- and 19-year-old siblings.[7] In 1925, John Percy Lockhart-Mummery established the polyposis registry at St. Mark's Hospital in London, England,[7] and in 1951, the American geneticist, Eldon J. Gardner, described what became known as Gardner's syndrome, consisting of colorectal adenomas, desmoid tumors, bone tumors (osteomas), and soft cyst-like surface tumors (epidermoid cysts, fibromas, and sebaceous cysts).[8] The first description of HNPCC was published in 1913, when Aldred Warthin, a University of Michigan pathologist, reported on "cancer family syndrome" kindreds, displaying multigenerational cancers of the colon, stomach, and uterus.[9] Additionally, he noted that these familial cancers were often diagnosed at young ages. In work that began in the 1960s, Henry Lynch followed cancer families, including Warthin's family G, and refined the definition of HNPCC into Lynch syndrome I, in which only colorectal cancer was diagnosed, and Lynch syndrome II, in which colorectal cancer in addition to extracolonic cancers, in particular endometrial cancer, were observed.[10] Transitional cell carcinoma of the ureter and renal pelvis and carcinomas of the stomach, small bowel, ovary, and pancreas were also present in Lynch syndrome II. Lynch observed that in these kindreds, colorectal cancer was diagnosed at an early age (average of 44 years) and that approximately 70% of these colorectal cancers arose proximal to splenic flexure. Clinically, HNPCC is defined by the International Collaborative Group on Hereditary Nonpolyposis Colorectal Cancer in terms of the following Amsterdam II criteria[11]:

1. Three or more relatives with HNPCC-associated cancer (colorectal, endometrial, stomach, ovary, ureter or renal pelvis, brain, small bowel, hepatobilairy tract cancers, or sebaceous tumors)
2. One affected individual should be a first-degree relative of the other two
3. Two or more successive generations should be affected
4. One or more of these cancers should be diagnosed before the age of 50 years
5. FAP should be excluded
6. Tumors should be verified by pathologic examination

The stepwise morphologic progression of colorectal neoplastic development and the accessibility of lesions at each stage of the progression have been key to the enormous growth in colorectal cancer molecular genetic knowledge over the past 30 years. The concept of adenoma to carcinoma progression was reported in the literature as early as the 1950s but gained broad interest with the studies of Basil Clifford Morson, in the 1960s and 1970s.[12] Morson surveyed more than 1000 pathology specimens, reporting the occurrence of malignant foci in large adenomas or residual benign adenoma adjacent to early colorectal cancers. Morson further noted the close histologic similarities between these adjacent invasive and noninvasive lesions. Studies have demonstrated an increased risk of colorectal cancer in individuals with polyps, and a reduction in cancer incidence can be achieved with systematic removal of benign adenomas.[13,14]

It is now firmly established that the morphologic stages of colorectal neoplastic progression include (1) aberrant crypt foci, which are very early colonic lesions, visible by methylene blue staining and microsopic examination without sectioning or histologic preparation[15]; (2) adenomas, which can be categorized as early, intermediate, and late (or I, II, and III), on the basis of increasing size, increasing villous component, and severity of dysplasia; and (3) invasive carcinomas, which can be categorized by histologic grade (differentiation) and pathologic stage of progression.

ADENOMA TO CARCINOMA: A GENETIC MODEL FOR COLORECTAL CARCINOGENESIS

From a molecular genetic standpoint, a cancer can be considered a clonal proliferation of cells characterized by autonomous growth and somatic heritable genetic alterations.[2] According to the theory of clonal selection, as a clone of altered cells proliferates (as in a very early small adenoma), random genetic alterations occur. When these alterations occur in genes that give the cell a growth advantage, this new subclone then expands preferentially. The new clone (a larger adenoma) then undergoes further genetic alterations and when these mutations cause a proliferative advantage they again will be selected. This process is continual over the lifetime of a neoplasm, resulting in the selection of multiple growth-advantageous mutations. Thus, tissue progresses from normal to adenomatous to invasive cancer by the accumulation and clonal expansion of a series of genetic alterations. A key implication of this theory is that most clonal somatic alterations detected in end-stage carcinomas should be important in having conferred growth advantage properties to the tumor.[16] In support of clonal origin from a single ancestral cell, all cells from the same colorectal cancer have been observed to share identical chromosome X inactivation (lyonization).[17] Furthermore, the ability to observe genetic mutations in bulk DNA preparations from colorectal cancers and adenomas implies that these mutations were present in the vast majority of the neoplastic cells being tested as a result of clonal selection during cancer progression.[5]

Direct genetic analysis has allowed observation of which gene alterations are involved in clonal colorectal cancer development and also has allowed study of the relative timing of these events. Some of the genetic alterations observed in colorectal neoplasms do occur in a preferred order and may directly relate to morphologic development. Each stage of this morphologic progression is associated with an increase in the total number of genetic alterations.[5] Furthermore, the temporal pattern of some genetic alterations suggests a critical role in the initiation or progression of colorectal neoplasia. For instance, studies suggest that the prevalence of APC gene inactivation is similar (more than 80%) at all stages of adenoma to carcinoma progression.[18] This suggests that APC gene inactivation is an early event in colorectal carcinogenesis and is further supported by the presence of APC gene mutations in dysplastic colorectal aberrant crypt foci but not in adjacent normal mucosa.[19]

Oncogenic K-ras gene mutations are also thought to occur as relatively early events in neoplastic progression.[5] These mutations are present in approximately 50% of intermediate stage adenomas and approximately 50% of carcinomas, suggesting their predominant occurrence in the early adenoma stage. The presence of K-ras, but not APC gene mutations, in a significant percentage of hyperplastic polyps and hyperplastic aberrant crypt foci, lesions not thought to have significant malignant potential, indirectly implicates mutation of APC, but not K-ras, as an initial genetic alteration in colorectal carcinogenesis.[5,19]

The presence of chromosome 17p allelic deletions usually occurs as a late event in colorectal carcinogenesis and corresponds to point mutations in the p53 gene.[5,20] Chromosome 17p loss is observed in 75% of carcinomas and 35% of late adenomas but only rarely in early adenomas. Similarly, the presence of chromosome 18q loss of heterozygosity also seems to be a late event in neoplastic progression and is observed in 10% of early adenomas, nearly 50% of late adenomas, and 70% of carcinomas.[5,21]

The frequent losses observed on chromosome 18q may relate to loss of function mutations of the DCC, SMAD4, or MADR2 genes.[21-23]

Taken together, these observations have led to the classical Vogelstein genetic model for colorectal tumorigenesis in which APC mutation and chromosome 5q loss followed by K-ras activation occur early in neoplasia intiation and adenoma formation, followed thereafter by p53 mutation, chromosome 17p loss, and additional loss of function alterations to chromosome 18q genetic targets later in colorectal progression from adenoma to carcinoma.[4,5]

CLASSES OF COLORECTAL CANCER GENES
Oncogenes and Tumor Suppressor Genes

Cancer genes are classified as oncogenes or tumor suppressor genes (antioncogenes) based on whether or not there is a gain or loss of wild-type genetic function in the cancer compared with the normal cells. Oncogenes were the first class of genes found associated with cancer and were identified in viruses that induced cancer in birds and rodents.[24] It was subsequently discovered that the genetic sequences responsible for this oncogenic transformation were stretches of normal DNA from former viral hosts, which the viruses had integrated into the host genome and were expressing aberrantly. These normal genes, known as proto-oncogenes, code for proteins involved in cell growth and differentiation. The consequence of proto-oncogene activation is abnormal proliferation of cells, in conditions where they would normally be quiescent or die. Mechanisms of activation include point mutation (ie, K-ras), gene amplification (ie, c-Myc), or chromosomal translocation (ie, BCR/ABL), all of which deregulate gene expression or create a chimeric protein with an abnormal function. Activating, somatic mutations of the receptor tyrosine kinase pathway genes, K-ras or BRAF, are observed commonly in colorectal cancers.[25-27] Mutations of one K-ras allele at codons 12, 13, and 61 account for more than 90% of the K-ras mutations observed in colorectal cancers and lead to a constitutively active protein, locked in its GTP-bound state.[4] BRAF acts downstream of K-ras and the vast majority of BRAF mutations observed in colorectal cancer consist of a single nucleotide substitution, V600E (previously named V599E).[27] Similarly, activating oncogenic mutations of serine-threonine phosphorylation sites in the CTNNB1 (β-catenin) gene may substitute for loss of function APC mutations in driving Wnt pathway overexpression in colorectal cancers.[28]

The concept of the tumor suppressor gene arose from Knudson's hypothesis with regards to the development of retinoblastoma.[29] Based on the early age of onset and bilaterality of inherited retinoblastoma, Knudson proposed that two key events (hits), each altering one copy (allele) of a critical gene, were responsible for the occurrence of this tumor. In colorectal and other inherited cancers, one mutant (inactivated) copy of tumor suppressor gene is inherited in the germline, and somatic inactivation of the remaining second copy results in cancer. Because only one somatic hit was required in addition to the inherited, germline mutation, tumors would arise at a young age and often in multiplicity. In contrast, sporadic carcinogenesis required inactivation of both wild-type copies of a given tumor suppressor gene by somatic alterations.

In general, one copy of a tumor suppressor gene is usually mutated by an intragenic event (a point mutation or a small frameshift deletion or insertion), whereas the second copy is often inactivated by deletion of a large chromosomal segment or even an entire chromosomal arm. Therefore, identification of a common region of chromosomal loss in tumors has been used as a marker to localize important tumor suppressor genes.

Many regions of allelic loss are commonly observed in colorectal cancers and approximately 4 to 5 chromosomal alleles are lost in most colorectal cancer specimens.[30] As discussed previously, colorectal cancer chromosomal losses at 5q and 17p have been linked to inactivation of the APC and p53 tumor suppressor genes,[20,31] whereas the frequent losses observed on chromosome 18q may relate to loss of function mutations of the DCC, SMAD4, or MADR2 genes.[21–23]

Gatekeepers, Caretakers, and Landscapers

In recent years, Kinzler and Vogelstein have suggested that cancer genes may be classified in terms of their ontologic roles as gatekeepers, caretakers, or landscapers.[32,33] Gatekeeper gene alteration occurs early in neoplasia and is the rate-limiting step in initiating dysplasia in a particular tissue. As discussed previously, APC gene inactivation is observed in more than 80% of early and late adenomas and invasive cancers.[18] Furthermore, APC gene mutations have been observed in dysplastic colorectal aberrant crypt foci,[19] and germline mutations of the APC gene are the underlying genetic cause of FAP.[31,34] Thus, the APC gene has been dubbed the gatekeeper of colorectal neoplasia and serves as the rate-limiting event for the development of adenomas.[32]

It is widely accepted that a significant number of genetic alterations are required for cancer initiation and progression.[4,5] Based on the fact that the basal spontaneous mutation rate of a cell could unlikely account for the number of genetic errors encountered in a cancer cell, Loeb postulated that defects in DNA replication or proofreading were a fundamental early requirement for multistage carcinogenesis.[35,36] Expanding on this notion, Kinzler and Vogelstein have termed cancer genes where dysfunction leads to a general increase in mutation rate as caretaker genes.[32] As discussed later, germline mutations in DNA mismatch repair, a class of caretaker genes, leads to HNPCC and deficiency in this proofreading system are observed in approximately 15% of sporadic colorectal cancers.[37–41] As a caretaker system, a deficiency in mismatch repair does not directly cause the malignant phenotype but instead leads to an increased mutation rate and secondarily to mutations in the genes that directly give rise to cancer initiation and progression.[32]

In addition to germline gatekeeper APC mutations associated with FAP, a second inherited genetic predisposition to colorectal adenomatous polyposis and cancer has recently been identified with inherited mutations of the MYH gene (MYH-associated polyposis [MAP]).[42–44] Similar to DNA mismatch repair, MYH acts a colorectal cancer caretaker gene and participates in a DNA proofreading system, known as base-excision repair. Mutations of the MYH gene and base-excision deficiency lead to specific somatic G:C to T:A transversion mutations of the gatekeeper APC gene.

In addition to caretaker genes, a second class of indirectly acting cancer genes is termed landscaper genes.[33] Landscaper alteration is postulated to change the local milieu of the tissue and provide a microenvironment that is more susceptible to the development of neoplasia. Colorectal cancers that arise in patients with the inherited hamartomatous polyp syndromes, Peutz-Jeghers syndrome, juvenile polyposis syndrome, and Cowden disease, are thus attributed to landscaper gene mutations. Peutz-Jeghers syndrome is associated with germline STK11 gene mutations.[45,46] Germline mutations of the SMAD4 or BMPR1A genes, both involved in transforming growth factor-beta signaling, lead to juvenile polyposis syndrome.[47,48] Finally, germline mutations of the PTEN gene have been identified in patients with Cowden disease.[49,50] Loss of function mutations of all these genes seem to lead directly to the development of clonal colorectal hamartomatous polyps. Unlike the caretaker gene class where the indirect mechanism of carcinogenesis is well understood, it remains unclear how hamartomatous stromal changes associated with landscaper dysfunction secondarily lead to neoplasia. Mechanisms of control via regulation of extracellular matrix proteins, cellular surface markers, cellular adhesion molecules, and growth factors are proposed.[51]

MUTATOR PATHWAYS IN COLORECTAL CANCER

In a general sense, genetic alterations in cancer have been observed to occur macroscopically as alterations in chromosome number and structure[30,52,53] and microscopically as nucleotide changes involving individual genes.[25,26] Similarly, both macro- and microoopigenetic alterations are observed in human cancers.[54,55] As discussed previously, basal mutation rates seem Insufficient to account for the 6000 to 11,000 somatic alterations experimentally estimated to be present in a colon cancer cell genome[56,57] and have prompted the hypothesis that widespread genomic (or epigenomic) instability is an essential early step in carcinogenesis.[35,36] The proposed inherent defect that makes cancer cells susceptible to genomic instability is often referred to as the mutator phenotype. There now seem to be at least three distinct mutator phenotype pathways in colorectal and other cancers—the microsatellite instability, the chromosomal instability, and the cytosine polyguanine (CpG) island methylator phenotype (CIMP) pathways.

Approximately 15% of sporadic colorectal cancers display a molecular phenotype, known as high-frequency microsatellite instability (MSI or MSI-H), also known as replication error positive.[32] This molecular hallmark arises due to a deficiency in a DNA replication proofreading system, known as mismatch repair.[11,32] Mismatch repair-deficiency causes mutations in short repetitive DNA repeats, known as microsatellites (ie, cytosine-adenine dinucleotide repeats [(CA)n] or adenine mononucleotide repeats [(A)n]). It is estimated that the human genome contains hundreds of thousands of microsatellite repeat DNA regions, largely in noncoding (intronic) regions.[58,59] Microsatellite regions are highly polymorphic; thus, microsatellite repeat numbers often differ between individuals but are the same in all cells of any single individual. MSI is apparent when the copy number of that particular microsatellite DNA region is different in a cancer compared with normal tissue from that same individual (ie, $[CA]_5$ versus $[CA]_4$). MSI-H is defined as instability in two or more of the five National Cancer Institute–recommended panels of microsatellite loci.[60] Although serving as signature of mismatch repair deficiency, mutations of microsatellite DNA generally have no direct functional consequence on the cell, unless the microsatellite is located in the coding region of a gene.[58,60]

To date, germline mutations in four mismatch repair genes, MLH1, MSH2, MSH6, and PMS2, have been reported to give rise to HNPCC.[37–40] The majority of HNPCC occurs due to MLH1 or MSH2 mutations. In contrast to genetic mutations observed in HNPCC, sporadic MSI colorectal cancers seem to arise due to an epigenetic (non-mutational) phenomenon causing mismatch repair-deficiency.[41] In the majority of sporadic MSI colorectal cancers, the MLH1 gene is transcriptionally silenced by CpG island promoter methylation.

The majority of colorectal cancers are aneuploid, consistent with a chromosomal instability pathway.[61] Cancers with chromosomal instability display predominantly large genetic alterations, such as chromosomal losses (loss of heterozygosity), amplifications, translocations, and rearrangements. Each of these large-scale chromosomal changes affects potentially hundreds of thousands of DNA bases. The microsatellite and chromosomal instability pathways seem to be mutually exclusive. Colorectal cancers are MSI, mismatch repair-deficient and near diploid, or microsatellite stable, mismatch repair-proficient, and aneuploid.[32]

As discussed previously, colorectal cancers have long been known to harbor widespread and frequent allelic losses at many chromosomal arms, notably 5q, 17p, and 18q.[4,5,30] Chromosomal instability is thought to arise early in colorectal neoplastic progression. Consistent with this hypothesis, loss of heterozygosity has been observed in dysplastic human colorectal aberrant crypt foci and minute adenomatous polyps.[5,62] In recent studies, using sensitive molecular techniques and microdissected or laser-captured specimens, several investigators have demonstrated that more than 85% of adenomatous polyps display insertions and deletions of genetic material ranging in size from hundreds of bases to entire chromosomal arms.[56,63,64]

Chromosomal instability is defined as an increased rate of loss or gain of large portions of chromosomes or whole chromosomes in cancer.[65] To date, a few studies have directly documented an increased dynamic rate of chromosomal alterations in aneuploid human colon cancer cells.[66,67] From these studies, chromosomal instability occurs in a genetically dominant fashion.[67]

The underlying cause of this mutator pathway is enigmatic. Many mechanisms could theoretically contribute to chromosomal instability, including deregulation of any of the following: mitotic and cell cycle checkpoints, telomere shortening and telomerase expression, centrosome number, double-strand break repair, kinetochore function, and chromatid separation.[67,68] Several mitotic spindle and cell cycle genes, such as BUB1, MAD2, Aurora A, and CDC4, seem to play a causative role in chromosomal instability in a modest subset of colorectal cancers with aneuploidy.[69–74]

There is mounting evidence that specific truncating mutations of the APC gene play a critical role in establishing chromosomal instability in the majority of colorectal adenomas and carcinomas.[75] Wild-type APC protein has been observed to physically associate with the mitotic spindle, and expression of truncated APC protein has been observed to produce high rates of karyotypic abnormalities.[76,77]

Hypermethylation of CpG islands in gene promoter regions is associated with loss of transcription and implicated as a nonmutational, epigenetic mechanism of gene inactivation in various human tumors.[78] A widespread nonrandom CIMP is identified in approximately 15% to 20% of colorectal cancers.[79,80] A five-marker panel to define CIMP-positive (CIMP+) colon cancer has been proposed and validated.[80,81] Consistent with a role promoting neoplasia, CIMP+ cancers frequently display epigenetic silencing of the p16 (cell cycle regulator), THBS1 (angiogenesis inhibitor) and MLH1 genes, and oncogenic BRAF point mutations.[79,80] Virtually all sporadic MSI colorectal cancers seem to arise in the context of CIMP+ and MLH1 silencing, whereas CIMP+ is never observed in HNPCC MSI cancers.[80] MLH1 silencing is not a constant event in CIMP+ cancers, however, and approximately 12% of microsatellite stable sporadic colorectal cancers also display CIMP+. Although increased expression of DNA methyltrasferases would be the obvious candidate cause of CIMP+, no consistent pattern of DNA methyltrasferase overexpression has been observed in CIMP+ colorectal cancers; thus, the underlying mechanism leading to the CIMP+ epigenetic mutator phenotype remains unresolved.[78]

SUMMARY

Cancer is fundamentally a genetic disease in which the clonal accumulation of genetic alterations confers a cell with the malignant characteristics of uncontrolled growth, local invasiveness, and metastatic potential. Studies of colorectal cancer and its precursor lesion, the adenomatous polyp, have served as the cornerstone in advancing knowledge of cancer molecular genetics. Although the origins of published cancer genetics dates back to more than 100 years ago, the past 30 years have ushered in an era of revolutionary increases in understanding colorectal cancer genetics. In the past few decades, many of the germline and somatic genetic events responsible for colorectal carcinogenesis have been identified, a model of the relative timing of the genetic events that cause adenoma to carcinoma progression developed, ontologic classification of cancer-causing genes defined, and distinct colorectal cancer mutator pathways elucidated. This knowledge has assisted in the ability to identify individuals at risk for developing colorectal cancer and has led to a better understanding of disease prognosis and response to therapy. In the future, it is hoped that the tremendous recent gains made in understanding of colorectal cancer genetics will allow for significant, tailored chemoprevention and treatment of this common malignancy.

REFERENCES

1. Jemal A, Siegel R, Ward E, et al. Cancer statistics, 2009. CA Cancer J Clin 2009; 59:225–49.
2. Nowell PC. The clonal evolution of tumor cell populations. Science 1976;194: 23–8.
3. Vogelstein B, Kinzler KW. Cancer genes and the pathways they control. Nat Med 2004;10:789–99.
4. Fearon ER, Vogelstein B. A genetic model for colorectal tumorigenesis. Cell 1990; 61:759–67.
5. Vogelstein B, Fearon ER, Hamilton SR, et al. Genetic alterations during colorectal-tumor development. N Engl J Med 1988;319:525–32.
6. Bignold LP, Coghlan BL, Jersmann HP. Hansemann, Boveri, chromosomes and the gametogenesis-related theories of tumours. Cell Biol Int 2006;30:640–4.
7. Bulow S, Berk T, Neale K. The history of familial adenomatous polyposis. Fam Cancer 2006;5:213–20.
8. Gardner EJ. A genetic and clinical study of intestinal polyposis, a predisposing factor for carcinoma of the colon and rectum. Am J Hum Genet 1951;3:167–76.
9. Lynch HT. Classics in oncology. Aldred Scott Warthin, M.D., Ph.D. (1866–1931). CA Cancer J Clin 1985;35:345–7.
10. Lynch HT, Smyrk TC, Watson P, et al. Genetics, natural history, tumor spectrum, and pathology of hereditary nonpolyposis colorectal cancer: an updated review. Gastroenterology 1993;104:1535–49.
11. Umar A, Boland CR, Terdiman JP, et al. Revised Bethesda guidelines for hereditary nonpolyposis colorectal cancer (Lynch syndrome) and microsatellite instability. J Natl Cancer Inst 2004;96:261–8.
12. Morson B. President's address. The polyp-cancer sequence in the large bowel. Proc R Soc Med 1974;67:451–7.
13. Atkin WS, Morson BC, Cuzick J. Long-term risk of colorectal cancer after excision of rectosigmoid adenomas. N Engl J Med 1992;326:658–62.
14. Winawer SJ, Zauber AG, Ho MN, et al. Prevention of colorectal cancer by colonoscopic polypectomy. The National Polyp Study Workgroup. N Engl J Med 1993; 329:1977–81.
15. Roncucci L, Stamp D, Medline A, et al. Identification and quantification of aberrant crypt foci and microadenomas in the human colon. Hum Pathol 1991;22: 287–94.

16. Kern SE. Clonality: more than just a tumor-progression model. J Natl Cancer Inst 1993;85:1020–1.
17. Vogelstein B, Fearon ER, Hamilton SR, et al. Clonal analysis using recombinant DNA probes from the X-chromosome. Cancer Res 1987;47:4806–13.
18. Powell SM, Zilz N, Beazer-Barclay Y, et al. APC mutations occur early during colorectal tumorigenesis. Nature 1992;359:235–7.
19. Smith AJ, Stern HS, Penner M, et al. Somatic APC and K-ras codon 12 mutations in aberrant crypt foci from human colons. Cancer Res 1994;54:5527–30.
20. Baker SJ, Fearon ER, Nigro JM, et al. Chromosome 17 deletions and p53 gene mutations in colorectal carcinomas. Science 1989;244:217–21.
21. Fearon ER, Cho KR, Nigro JM, et al. Identification of a chromosome 18q gene that is altered in colorectal cancers. Science 1990;247:49–56.
22. Hahn SA, Schutte M, Hoque AT, et al. DPC4, a candidate tumor suppressor gene at human chromosome 18q21.1. Science 1996;271:350–3.
23. Eppert K, Scherer SW, Ozcelik H, et al. MADR2 maps to 18q21 and encodes a TGFbeta-regulated MAD-related protein that is functionally mutated in colorectal carcinoma. Cell 1996;86:543–52.
24. McLaughlin-Drubin ME, Munger K. Viruses associated with human cancer. Biochim Biophys Acta 2008;1782:127–50.
25. Bos JL, Fearon ER, Hamilton SR, et al. Prevalence of ras gene mutations in human colorectal cancers. Nature 1987;327:293–7.
26. Forrester K, Almoguera C, Han K, et al. Detection of high incidence of K-ras oncogenes during human colon tumorigenesis. Nature 1987;327:298–303.
27. Rajagopalan H, Bardelli A, Lengauer C, et al. Tumorigenesis: RAF/RAS oncogenes and mismatch-repair status. Nature 2002;418:934.
28. Morin PJ, Sparks AB, Korinek V, et al. Activation of beta-catenin-Tcf signaling in colon cancer by mutations in beta-catenin or APC. Science 1997;275:1787–90.
29. Knudson AG Jr. Mutation and cancer: statistical study of retinoblastoma. Proc Natl Acad Sci U S A 1971;68:820–3.
30. Vogelstein B, Fearon ER, Kern SE, et al. Allelotype of colorectal carcinomas. Science 1989;244:207–11.
31. Nishisho I, Nakamura Y, Miyoshi Y, et al. Mutations of chromosome 5q21 genes in FAP and colorectal cancer patients. Science 1991;253:665–9.
32. Kinzler KW, Vogelstein B. Lessons from hereditary colorectal cancer. Cell 1996; 87:159–70.
33. Kinzler KW, Vogelstein B. Landscaping the cancer terrain. Science 1998;280: 1036–7.
34. Kinzler KW, Nilbert MC, Su LK, et al. Identification of FAP locus genes from chromosome 5q21. Science 1991;253:661–5.
35. Loeb LA, Springgate CF, Battula N. Errors in DNA replication as a basis of malignant changes. Cancer Res 1974;34:2311–21.
36. Loeb LA. Mutator phenotype may be required for multistage carcinogenesis. Cancer Res 1991;51:3075–9.
37. Fishel R, Lescoe MK, Rao MR, et al. The human mutator gene homolog MSH2 and its association with hereditary nonpolyposis colon cancer. Cell 1993;75: 1027–38.
38. Leach FS, Nicolaides NC, Papadopoulos N, et al. Mutations of a mutS homolog in hereditary nonpolyposis colorectal cancer. Cell 1993;75:1215–25.
39. Bronner CE, Baker SM, Morrison PT, et al. Mutation in the DNA mismatch repair gene homologue hMLH1 is associated with hereditary non-polyposis colon cancer. Nature 1994;368:258–61.

40. Nicolaides NC, Papadopoulos N, Liu B, et al. Mutations of two PMS homologues in hereditary nonpolyposis colon cancer. Nature 1994;371:75–80.
41. Kane MF, Loda M, Gaida GM, et al. Methylation of the hMLH1 promoter correlates with lack of expression of hMLH1 in sporadic colon tumors and mismatch repair-defective human tumor cell lines. Cancer Res 1997;57:808–11.
42. Al-Tassan N, Chmiel NH, Maynard J, et al. Inherited variants of MYH associated with somatic G: C–T: a mutations in colorectal tumors. Nat Genet 2002;30:227–32.
43. Sieber OM, Lipton L, Crabtree M, et al. Multiple colorectal adenomas, classic adenomatous polyposis, and germ-line mutations in MYH. N Engl J Med 2003; 348:791–9.
44. Croitoru ME, Cleary SP, Di Nicola N, et al. Association between biallelic and monoallelic germline MYH gene mutations and colorectal cancer risk. J Natl Cancer Inst 2004;96:1631–4.
45. Hemminki A, Markie D, Tomlinson I, et al. A serine/threonine kinase gene defective in Peutz-Jeghers syndrome. Nature 1998;391:184–7.
46. Jenne DE, Reimann H, Nezu J, et al. Peutz-Jeghers syndrome is caused by mutations in a novel serine threonine kinase. Nat Genet 1998;18:38–43.
47. Howe JR, Roth S, Ringold JC, et al. Mutations in the SMAD4/DPC4 gene in juvenile polyposis. Science 1998;280:1086–8.
48. Howe JR, Bair JL, Sayed MG, et al. Germline mutations of the gene encoding bone morphogenetic protein receptor 1A in juvenile polyposis. Nat Genet 2001; 28:184–7.
49. Marsh DJ, Dahia PL, Zheng Z, et al. Germline mutations in PTEN are present in Bannayan-Zonana syndrome. Nat Genet 1997;16:333–4.
50. Liaw D, Marsh DJ, Li J, et al. Germline mutations of the PTEN gene in Cowden disease, an inherited breast and thyroid cancer syndrome. Nat Genet 1997;16: 64–7.
51. Macleod K. Tumor suppressor genes. Curr Opin Genet Dev 2000;10:81–93.
52. Boveri T. Zur Frage der Entstehung maligner Tumoren [On the question of the origin of malignant tumors.]. Jena, Germany: Gustav Fischer Verlag; 1914 [in German].
53. Law DJ, Olschwang S, Monpezat JP, et al. Concerted nonsyntenic allelic loss in human colorectal carcinoma. Science 1988;241:961–5.
54. Goelz SE, Vogelstein B, Hamilton SR, et al. Hypomethylation of DNA from benign and malignant human colon neoplasms. Science 1985;228:187–90.
55. Greger V, Passarge E, Hopping W, et al. Epigenetic changes may contribute to the formation and spontaneous regression of retinoblastoma. Hum Genet 1989; 83:155–8.
56. Stoler DL, Chen N, Basik M, et al. The onset and extent of genomic instability in sporadic colorectal tumor progression. Proc Natl Acad Sci U S A 1999;96: 15121–6.
57. Wang TL, Rago C, Silliman N, et al. Prevalence of somatic alterations in the colorectal cancer cell genome. Proc Natl Acad Sci U S A 2002;99:3076–80.
58. Ionov Y, Peinado MA, Malkhosyan S, et al. Ubiquitous somatic mutations in simple repeated sequences reveal a new mechanism for colonic carcinogenesis. Nature 1993;363:558–61.
59. Thibodeau SN, Bren G, Schaid D. Microsatellite instability in cancer of the proximal colon. Science 1993;260:816–9.
60. Boland CR, Thibodeau SN, Hamilton SR, et al. National Cancer Institute Workshop on Microsatellite Instability for cancer detection and familial

predisposition: development of international criteria for the determination of microsatellite instability in colorectal cancer. Cancer Res 1998;58:5248–57.

61. Goh HS, Jass JR. DNA content and the adenoma-carcinoma sequence in the colorectum. J Clin Pathol 1986;39:387–92.

62. Luo L, Shen GQ, Stiffler KA, et al. Loss of heterozygosity in human aberrant crypt foci (ACF), a putative precursor of colon cancer. Carcinogenesis 2006;27: 1153–9.

63. Shih IM, Zhou W, Goodman SN, et al. Evidence that genetic instability occurs at an early stage of colorectal tumorigenesis. Cancer Res 2001;61:818–22.

64. Cardoso J, Molenaar L, de Menezes RX, et al. Chromosomal instability in MYH- and APC-mutant adenomatous polyps. Cancer Res 2006;66:2514–9.

65. Rajagopalan H, Nowak MA, Vogelstein B, et al. The significance of unstable chromosomes in colorectal cancer. Nat Rev Cancer 2003;3:695–701.

66. Phear G, Bhattacharyya NP, Meuth M. Loss of heterozygosity and base substitution at the APRT locus in mismatch-repair-proficient and -deficient colorectal carcinoma cell lines. Mol Cell Biol 1996;16:6516–23.

67. Lengauer C, Kinzler KW, Vogelstein B. Genetic instability in colorectal cancers. Nature 1997;386:623–7.

68. Wang Z, Cummins JM, Shen D, et al. Three classes of genes mutated in colorectal cancers with chromosomal instability. Cancer Res 2004;64:2998–3001.

69. Cahill DP, Lengauer C, Yu J, et al. Mutations of mitotic checkpoint genes in human cancers. Nature 1998;392:300–3.

70. Michel LS, Liberal V, Chatterjee A, et al. MAD2 haplo-insufficiency causes premature anaphase and chromosome instability in mammalian cells. Nature 2001;409:355–9.

71. Bischoff JR, Anderson L, Zhu Y, et al. A homologue of Drosophila aurora kinase is oncogenic and amplified in human colorectal cancers. EMBO J 1998;17: 3052–65.

72. Zhou H, Kuang J, Zhong L, et al. Tumour amplified kinase STK15/BTAK induces centrosome amplification, aneuploidy and transformation. Nat Genet 1998;20: 189–93.

73. Rajagopalan H, Jallepalli PV, Rago C, et al. Inactivation of hCDC4 can cause chromosomal instability. Nature 2004;428:77–81.

74. Akhoondi S, Sun D, von der Lehr N, et al. FBXW7/hCDC4 is a general tumor suppressor in human cancer. Cancer Res 2007;67:9006–12.

75. Pellman D. Cancer. A CINtillating new job for the APC tumor suppressor. Science 2001;291:2555–6.

76. Kaplan KB, Burds AA, Swedlow JR, et al. A role for the adenomatous polyposis coli protein in chromosome segregation. Nat Cell Biol 2001;3:429–32.

77. Fodde R, Kuipers J, Rosenberg C, et al. Mutations in the APC tumour suppressor gene cause chromosomal instability. Nat Cell Biol 2001;3:433–8.

78. Teodoridis JM, Hardie C, Brown R. CpG island methylator phenotype (CIMP) in cancer: causes and implications. Cancer Lett 2008;268:177–86.

79. Toyota M, Ahuja N, Ohe-Toyota M, et al. CpG island methylator phenotype in colorectal cancer. Proc Natl Acad Sci U S A 1999;96:8681–6.

80. Weisenberger DJ, Siegmund KD, Campan M, et al. CpG island methylator phenotype underlies sporadic microsatellite instability and is tightly associated with BRAF mutation in colorectal cancer. Nat Genet 2006;38:787–93.

81. Ogino S, Kawasaki T, Kirkner GJ, et al. Evaluation of markers for CpG island methylator phenotype (CIMP) in colorectal cancer by a large population-based sample. J Mol Diagn 2007;9:305–14.

Familial Adenomatous Polyposis

James Church, MB, ChB, FRACS

KEYWORDS

• Familial • Adenomatous • Polyposis • Surgery

Familial adenomatous polyposis (FAP) is a dominantly inherited syndrome of colorectal cancer predisposition owing to a germline mutation in the *APC* gene. Although it is rare (1 in 8000 to 12,000 live births), FAP is important for the health and lifestyle of affected patients and their families and also for what it can teach us about colorectal carcinogenesis in general. The broad term "Familial adenomatous polyposis" includes several subcategories of subtly different variants (see **Table 1**), but all these variants share a germline *APC* mutation as their etiology. The syndrome can be defined phenotypically (see **Table 1**) or genotypically. The problem with a genotypic definition is that some patients with FAP may not have a detectable germline mutation, or may have a mutation or deletion that is hard to detect.

Differential diagnosis of mild and classical FAP includes hyperplastic polyposis, lymphoid polyposis, and inflammatory polyposis. These conditions are easily separated from FAP by biopsy of a representative number of polyps. Differential diagnosis of attenuated FAP includes MYH-associated polyposis, a recessively inherited syndrome of colorectal cancer predisposition due to biallelic mutations in the base excision repair gene *MYH*.[2,3]

HISTORY

The first definite cases of adenomatous polyposis involved a 16-year-old girl and a 21-year-old man, reported by Chargelaigue in 1859.[4] In 1882, Cripps described a familial pattern of colorectal polyposis in a 9-year-old boy and his 17-year-old sister.[5] Eight years later multiple rectal polyps were described in succeeding generations.[6] The foundations of our modern treatment of FAP were laid at St Marks Hospital in London England, where Lockhart Mummery established the first FAP registry. However it was the pathology lab assistant, Basil Morson, who developed a keen interest in the syndrome and facilitated an understanding of the pathogenesis of colorectal cancer in FAP. Surgery for FAP was first described in the early twentieth century,

Department of Colorectal Surgery, Sanford R. Weiss Center for Hereditary Colorectal Neoplasia, Digestive Diseases Institute, Cleveland Clinic Foundation, 9500 Euclid Ave, Desk A30, Cleveland, OH 44195, USA
E-mail address: churchj@ccf.org

Surg Oncol Clin N Am 18 (2009) 585–598
doi:10.1016/j.soc.2009.07.002
1055-3207/09/$ – see front matter © 2009 Elsevier Inc. All rights reserved.

Table 1	
Definitions of familial adenomatous polyposis	
Variant	**Definition**
Attenuated familial polyposis[1]	<100 synchronous colorectal adenomas
Mild polyposis	100 to 1000 synchronous colorectal adenomas
Severe (profuse) polyposis	> 1000 synchronous colorectal adenomas
Gardner's syndrome	FAP with the following extracolonic manifestations: osteomas, epidermoid cysts, extra teeth, desmoid disease
Turcot's syndrome	FAP with medulloblastoma (astrocytoma)

Abbreviation: FAP, familial adenomatous polyposis.

by J.P. Lockhart-Mummery in England at St Marks Hospital and Lilienthal in the United States.[7] Prophylactic colectomy and ileorectal anastomosis became the procedure of choice and has successfully prevented cancer in many affected patients. In the early 1980s, total proctocolectomy and ileo-anal pouch anastomosis became popular for severe polyposis.

Technical advances in gastroenterology, surgery, and molecular biology have been applied to FAP and have proven valuable. Flexible endoscopy, arriving in the 1960s, allowed routine surveillance of the stomach, duodenum, and large bowel. APC was cloned in 1991[8] and techniques for detecting mutations developed from linkage analysis to protein truncation testing and now, sequencing. Minimally invasive surgery is the latest technical advance to benefit patients with FAP.

Other, nontechnical advances have had an even greater impact on the lives of patients with polyposis. Lockhart-Mummery and his colleagues at St Marks Hospital set the precedent for the registration and organized screening of patients at risk, and so showed the benefits of a Polyposis Registry. International collaboration between registries and centers is currently manifest in the International Society for Gastrointestinal Hereditary Tumors (InSiGHT) and the Collaborative Group of the Americas on Inherited Colorectal Cancer (CGA-ICC). In 2009 our level of knowledge about FAP is at an all-time high. Of course there is more to learn, and we still await practical gene therapy as a way of avoiding the phenotypic manifestations of disease altogether. A more immediate priority, however, is to ensure that the current level of knowledge is widely available, so that all affected patients and families have access to scientifically based, appropriate therapy, regardless where they live.

INCIDENCE AND EPIDEMIOLOGY

The incidence of FAP is estimated at 1 in 10,000 live births. Prevalence is about 1 in 24,000. Most doctors will at most see only a handful of cases, unless they practice in a specialized unit or tertiary referral center.

As expected from an autosomal dominant disease, FAP affects both genders and all races, although the expression of the disease may vary. Desmoid tumors, for example, tend to behave worst in young, nulliparous women and affect women twice as frequently as men. Similarly, the range of diseases associated with a germline APC mutation may vary from one country or lifestyle to another. The incidence of gastric cancer is higher in Japan than in Western countries, with the incidence in Korea somewhere between Japan and the West.[9,10]

GENETICS

FAP is an autosomal, dominantly Inherited syndrome of cancer predisposition owing to a germline mutation in APC. Dominant, autosomal inheritance is well seen in a typical family tree such as is shown in **Fig. 1**.

APC is an important "gatekeeper" gene involved in the key Wnt/Wingless growth regulation pathway.[11] More than 840 different APC mutations have been described, encompassing the entire length of the gene. Most cause a truncated APC protein, reducing the "dose" of normal APC within the cell. When the function of the remaining normal allele is lost, either by a (somatic) mutation, loss of heterozygosity, or decrease in expression, β catenin is able to enter the nucleus and trigger downstream pathways of cellular proliferation.

The germline APC mutation underlying FAP is highly penetrant; 100% penetrance means that all carriers of a germline mutation are guaranteed to develop the disease. The phenotype (the clinical manifestations) associated with the genotype (the site of the mutation within the gene) varies however, and depends in part on the location of the mutation. Commonly observed phenotype/genotype associations are shown in **Fig. 2**. They allow prediction of polyposis severity and desmoid risk, and explain the finding of congenital hypertrophy of the retinal pigmented epithelium (CHRPE) in 66% of FAP families. Genotype/phenotype predictions are not exact, however, as in many FAP families (each family member with the same mutation) there are variations in disease pattern. These intrafamilial variations may be attributable to modifier genes or environmental influences, and represent one of the major current puzzles in FAP science.

GENETIC TESTING

The best way of diagnosing FAP in an at-risk individual and to screen for FAP in a family is by genetic testing. DNA, usually obtained from blood leucocytes, is sequenced looking for mutations in the coding sequence of the gene. An affected patient (who clinically has FAP) is tested first. If a pathologic mutation is found, then the at-risk members in the family can be tested. If a mutation is not found, techniques such as conversion analysis or Southern blotting can be used to test for large deletions.[12] If no APC mutation is found, the DNA can be tested for bilallelic MYH mutations. If no mutation is found, the at-risk family members must be screened with flexible sigmoidoscopy (classic or profuse polyposis) or colonoscopy (attenuated polyposis).

Genetic counseling is a prerequisite to genetic testing, so that the patient and family can be acquainted with the implications of genetic testing, and can understand how and why it is helpful. Genetic counseling includes education about the syndrome, essential to understanding the surgical options, the need for surveillance, and the consequences of noncompliance.[13]

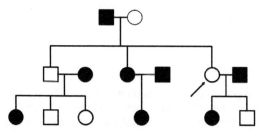

Fig. 1. Family tree representing dominant inheritance. Open square, affected male; closed square, unaffected male; open circle, affected female; closed circle, unaffected female.

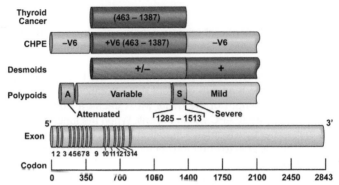

Fig. 2. Genotype-phenotype association with germline *APC* mutations in familial adenoma tous polyposis.

PRESENTATION

Patients affected with FAP present without symptoms, either on screening or serendipitously during investigation of some unrelated complaint, or with symptoms because they escaped screening. The commonest reason for failure to screen is that there is no family history. One quarter of patients with FAP have no family history, usually because they have a "de novo" mutation.[14] Other reasons for the lack of a family history include adoption, lack of knowledge, and a deliberate withholding of knowledge by family members. Without a positive family history there is no warning of risk and the polyposis develops until symptoms occur. When symptoms occur, more than 60% of patients have a colorectal cancer.[15] Screening, either by genetic testing or flexible endoscopy, can prevent almost all of these cancers.

Symptoms suggestive of polyposis include rectal bleeding, altered bowl habit, and abdominal pain. These are normally investigated by endoscopy and multiple polyps are seen. Representative biopsies confirm the diagnosis of adenomatous polyps.

Screening normally begins at puberty, the age at which therapeutic decisions begin to be clinically relevant. If genetic screening is not possible, flexible sigmoidoscopy can be done. If polyps are seen they are biopsied, and if they are adenomatous, colonoscopy is scheduled to assess the severity of the disease. If genetic screening shows that a child carries a mutation, yearly colonoscopy is begun.

Sometimes extracolonic manifestations of the *APC* mutation prompt referral for genetic testing and colonoscopy. An alert dentist will refer a patient with extra teeth seen on panorex examination, a dermatologist may refer for osteomas or epidermoid cysts, an ophthalmologist may refer for congenital hypertrophy of the retinal pigment epithelium (CHRPE), and a surgeon may refer for intra-abdominal desmoids.

EXTRACOLONIC MANIFESTATIONS

FAP is the result of a germline *APC* mutation, and as such is manifest by benign and malignant tumors in a variety of organs. These are listed in **Table 2**. The most common manifestations are gastric fundic gland polyps and duodenal adenomas, found in more than 90% of patients. The association of polyposis with osteomas, epidermoid cysts, extra teeth, and desmoid tumors has been referred to as Gardner's syndrome.

Table 2
Manifestations of a germline familial adenomatous polyposis mutation

Organ	Benign	Malignant
Skin	Epidermoid cyst	
Bone	Osteoma	
Stomach	Fundic gland polyp Adenoma	Adenocarcinoma
Duodenum	Adenoma	Adenocarcinoma
Small bowel	Adenoma	Adenocarcinoma
Ileostomy	Adenoma	Adenocarcinoma
Thyroid		Papillary carcinoma
Adrenal	Adenoma	Adenocarcinoma
Liver		Hepatoblastoma
Brain		Medulloblastoma
Fibrous tissue	Desmoids	
Retina	Congenital hypertrophy of retinal pigmented epithelium	

WORK-UP

Patients newly diagnosed with FAP undergo colonoscopy to assess the number and distribution of adenomas. Note is made of any polyps that are fragile enough, irregular enough, and fixed enough to suggest cancer. This is especially important in the rectum, where rectal cancer radiation is often advised before a pouch-anal anastomosis. Patients older than 20 undergo esophago-gastro-duodenoscopy (EGD) with end and side-viewing scopes. A thorough clinical examination includes inspection for extracolonic manifestations. Thyroid screening is by ultrasound. Work-up can be guided by genotype and family history, especially for desmoid disease where a preoperative CT scan and preoperative desmoid prophylaxis may be considered.

COLORECTAL SURGERY

Patients with FAP will develop colorectal cancer at a median age of 39 years without surgery; prophylactic colectomy or proctocolectomy. The issues with prophylactic colorectal surgery in FAP are those of the choice of operation and the timing of operation. The goals are first to prevent colorectal cancer and second to maintain quality of life. This second aim is important, especially when the patient is a young adult in the most important developmental years of their life. These patients, usually asymptomatic, need a procedure with a low risk of complications, minimal impact on bowel function, and minimal disturbance of lifestyle. Balanced against this is the need to minimize the risk of cancer. The surgical options are four: colectomy with ileorectal anastomosis (IRA), proctocolectomy with ileal-pouch anal anastomosis (IPAA), proctocolectomy with ileostomy, and proctocolectomy with continent ileostomy. Advantages and disadvantages, indications and contraindications are shown in **Table 3**.

Colectomy with Ileorectal Anastomosis

Triaging the fate of the rectum according to the number, size, and histology of rectal polyps is effective in minimizing the need for future proctectomy. If there are fewer than 20 adenomas, none larger than 1 cm and none severely dysplastic, the rectum may be retained.[16] The IRA preserves excellent bowel function, is simple, and can be done laparoscopically with major benefits to the lifestyle of patients.[17]

Table 3
Options for colorectal surgery in patients with familial adenomatous polyposis

Option	Indications	Contraindications	Advantages	Disadvantages
Ileorectal anastomosis	<20 rectal adenomas <1000 colonic adenomas[16]	Severe dysplasia in the rectum Cancer anywhere in large bowel Large (>3cm) rectal adenomas	Avoids pelvic dissection Simple surgery Low complications Good functional result[17] No stoma	Retained rectum may need to be removed later Possibility of rectal cancer if patient is not compliant with follow-up
Ileal Pouch-anal anastomosis, stapled	>20 rectal adenomas, >1000 colonic adenomas[16] Severe dysplasia in the rectum Cancer anywhere in large bowel Large (>3 cm) rectal adenomas ATZ clear of adenomas	Incompetent sphincters Rectal cancer invading sphincters Pouch won't reach anus	Avoids permanent stoma Good function in most patients[18]	Higher complication rate May provoke desmoids Decreased ability to conceive in women.[19] Retained anal and low rectal mucosa may develop neoplasia (28%)[20]
Ileal Pouch-anal anastomosis, mucosectomy	>20 rectal adenomas, >1000 colonic adenomas[16] Severe dysplasia in the rectum Cancer anywhere in large bowel Large (>3 cm) rectal adenomas ATZ contains adenomas	Incompetent sphincters Rectal cancer invading sphincters Pouch won't reach anus	Avoids permanent stoma Reasonable function in most patients. No residual anal mucosa (although neoplasia can still occur)[18,20]	Highest complication rate May provoke desmoids Decreased ability to conceive in women[19] Frequent seepage Nighttime incontinence.[18] Anal neoplasia in 14%[20]
Proctocolectomy and ileostomy	>20 rectal adenomas, >1000 colonic adenomas Severe dysplasia in the rectum Cancer anywhere in large bowel Large (>3 cm) rectal adenomas ATZ contains adenomas Incompetent sphincters Rectal cancer invading sphincters Pouch won't reach anus	Competent sphincters No rectal cancer Pouch reaches anus	Low complication rate Low chance of reoperation No anal incontinence	Permanent stoma

Abbreviation: ATZ, anal transition zone.

An IRA can be defined as removal of the entire colon, leaving 15 cm of rectum for optimal bowel function.

Technical points of an IRA are:

1. Preoperative colonoscopy to assess the risk of a cancer. If there is no cancer, mesenteric resection may be reasonably conservative. If there are large suspicious polyps, mesenteric resection must be radical.
2. Rectal polyps larger than 1.0 cm are removed either preoperatively or intraoperatively and sent for permanent or frozen section to exclude rectal cancer. If there is cancer, the surgery can be changed to IPAA.
3. Resect the terminal ileum as it flares at the entry to the cecum, giving a wider lumen for the anastomosis.
4. Make sure the distal resection line is in the rectum.
5. If there is any suspicion of cancer in the colon, remove the omentum en bloc.
6. An ileorectal anastomosis may be more prone to leak than other enteric anastomoses. This may be because of disproportion in the size of bowel ends. Our preference is an end-to-end handsewn anastomosis, using a Cheatle slit in the ileum if necessary.
7. The mesenteric defect between the terminal ileum and the sacral promontory should be closed to prevent a small bowel hernia. A flap of ileal mesentery can be preserved to make this closure easy and under no tension.
8. Open the specimen before the abdomen is closed or the patient wakes. There may be a cancer that was not diagnosed preoperatively, and a more extensive mesenteric resection may be needed.

Postoperatively

If an IRA is done with minimally invasive technique the postoperative recovery usually involves a hospital stay of 2 to 4 days. Patients usually have two to four stools a day with good continence and minimal urgency.[17] Patients must understand that yearly proctoscopy is essential to monitor the growth of adenomas.

Surveillance of the rectum after IRA demands a good view (two enemas and flexible endoscopy). In long-standing IRAs after multiple polyp coagulations, rectal cancer can be flat and hard to detect, showing up as a red "patch" and analogous to the low-profile cancers seen in ulcerative colitis. Rectal polyps can be resected at the time of the IRA, but even if they are not, they tend to regress during the first 3 years postoperatively.[21] When polyps start to grow, small (<5 mm) lesions can be ignored whereas large (>5 mm) are snared. Chemoprophylaxis with sulindac or celebrex will minimize adenoma growth but will not necessarily prevent cancer.[22] It can be reserved for patients with significant polyp burden but who are not ready or suitable for proctectomy.

Trigger for proctectomy after IRA is an increasing instability of the rectal mucosa as evidenced by increasing polyp size or number. Severe dysplasia is also an indication, as is invasive cancer. In most cases, proctectomy and IPAA can be done although occasionally an IPAA is not possible because of inadequate bowel length or mesenteric desmoid tumors. The function of an IPAA after an IRA is similar to that of a de novo pouch.[23,24]

Proctocolectomy with Ileal-pouch Anal Anastomosis

Removal of the entire colon and rectum, down to the pelvic floor, achieves prevention of both colon and rectal cancer but requires construction of an ileal pouch. The "pouch" decreases stool frequency from more than 20 bowel movements per day with a straight ileo-anal anastomosis, to an average of 5 to 6. It works by creating a length of bowel with double the lumen and with no net peristaltic propulsion, stool emptying by gravity with no urgency. The key factors determining stool frequency are therefore pouch length and stool consistency. An anastomosis between an ileal pouch and the upper anus is performed. There are three options for the surgeon that affect the conduct of the operation: the type of pouch, the type of anastomosis, and construction of a diverting ileostomy.

Type of pouch

The most common and easiest pouch to make is the J pouch. Limbs are 15 to 20 cm long but the main factor determining length is the position of the apex of the superior mesenteric artery. The stool frequency of the J pouch is similar to an S pouch, made with three 15-cm limbs. The S pouch takes longer to make than the J, as it is hand-sewn, not stapled.

Type of anastomosis

The simpler type of anastomosis is a double-stapled end of pouch to anus anastomosis. The rectum is stapled distally at the level of the pelvic floor, a purse string suture is inserted into the open end of the pouch and used to tie in the anvil of the stapler, and the anastomosis is completed by transanal insertion of the stapler cartridge, uniting the cartridge with the anvil, and firing the stapler. Residual anal transition zone is often less than 1.0 cm, as the stapler removes 0.5 to 1.0 cm. Alternatively, the anal transition zone is stripped transanally (mucosectomy) and the pouch pulled into the anus and anastomosed by hand transanally to the dentate line. The stripping and hand-sewn anastomosis takes longer and in some studies is associated with more complications and worse function than the stapled anastomosis,[25] but its putative advantage is removal of all anal transitional and rectal epithelium with more complete prevention of anal transitional neoplasia.[18] However, anal transition zone cancers have been described after mucosectomy.[26] The prime indication for mucosectomy and handsewn IPAA is carpeting of the anal transitional zone by adenoma.

The anatomy of the pouch and the anus suggests that a J pouch is best suited to a stapled anastomosis at the top of the anal canal, and an S pouch to a handsewn anastomosis within the anus to the dentate line.

Diversion or no diversion

The IPAA was initially intended for use in patients with ulcerative colitis, who are often taking steroids or immunosuppressives, and have an inflamed large bowel. A diverting ileostomy is a routine part of an IPAA for such patients, because of a leak rate of at least 6% at the anastomosis and because of the inflamed anal transition zone (ATZ) to which the pouch is anastomosed. Over time, however, diversion has become optional in patients at low risk for an anastomotic complication. Patients with FAP are at low risk for an anastomotic leak or fistula because they are generally healthy, are not taking immunosuppressive medications, and have normal bowel except for the adenomas. Although an ileostomy creates the need for another surgery to close the ileostomy with its own risks of postoperative complications, an undiverted pouch is at a higher risk of anastomotic leak.[27] Therefore, in most patients a "safety first" approach is better and the postoperative course is smoother. In the short term, function of a freshly constructed pouch is worse than that of a healed pouch, and the postoperative ileus after construction of an undirected pouch can last several days.

The technical points of IPAA are as follows:

1. Preoperative colonoscopy is important to assess the risk of cancer. If it is clear that there is no cancer, mesenteric resection may be conservative. If there are any

adenomas larger than 1.0 cm, or any that look suspicious, mesenteric resection must be radical, the vessels taken close to their origin.

2. Rectal cancers should be carefully staged preoperatively and neoadjuvant chemo-radiation given for node-positive and advanced T3 lesions. Postoperative radiation after an IPAA may lead to such bad pouch dysfunction as to require pouch removal.

3. Make a judgment about the reach of the pouch before rectal dissection begins. If the apex of the superior mesenteric artery reaches below the symphysis pubis then a stapled IPAA will be possible; however, too much tension on the anastomosis predisposes to anastomotic separation.

4. Ways to extend the length of the small bowel mesentery include preserving the ileocolic arcade and dividing the superior mesenteric arcade at the tip of the pouch, making stepwise incisions in the peritoneum over the superior mesenteric artery, and making an S pouch instead of a J.

5. If there is any suspicion of cancer in the colon, remove the omentum en bloc.

6. Open the specimen, either in the operating room or the pathology laboratory, and examine it before the abdomen is closed or the patient wakes. There may be a hard area suggesting cancer and a more extensive mesenteric resection may be needed.

Postoperatively

If an IPAA is done with minimally invasive technique, the postoperative recovery is usually smooth, requiring a hospital stay of 3 to 5 days. After ileostomy closure, bowel function settles down over a few weeks to four to six stools a day, continence is good, and urgency is minimal. Yearly pouchoscopy is essential to monitor the growth of adenomas.

Pouch adenomas are not surprising, considering the combination of fecal stasis, a germline *APC* mutation, and rapidly turning over epithelium. The incidence of pouch adenomas is time-dependent, with 42% of patients affected at 7 years from pouch construction.[28] Pouch adenomas respond to Sulindac, but severe pouch polyposis may require pouchectomy.[26]

Indications, advantages, and disadvantages of IRA and IPAA for FAP are shown in **Table 3**.

FACTORS INFLUENCING CHOICE AND TIMING OF SURGERY

The most important consideration in the management of patients with FAP is to prevent cancer. Decisions regarding timing and type of surgery are made with this in mind. Preoperative assessment of genotype, phenotype, and family aims to estimate the risk of cancer being present and the timeline of its likely development. Thus, symptomatic patients need immediate surgery because of the chance of cancer already being present.[15] Asymptomatic patients can delay surgery as long as colonoscopy can rule out a cancer or a severely dysplastic polyp. Cancer is rare in patients younger than 20[29] and the ideal time for surgery is when patients have attained physical, mental, and social maturity, usually during late teenage years. With minimally invasive approaches, the disability associated with convalescence is minimal so that there is much less interruption of school or work. Financial concerns can guide timing of surgery, depending on coverage, deductibles, and other issues. A summary of timing advice is shown in **Table 4**. The determinants of the type of surgery are summarized in **Table 3**. The severity of polyposis remains the main factor driving the choice of surgery. Sometimes predictors of a bad outcome from pouch surgery such as extreme obesity or lax anal sphincters, or a patient's wish to avoid the decreased fecundity that is associated with IPAA, mean that a compromise approach

Table 4	
Timing of prophylactic colorectal surgery in familial adenomatous polyposis	
Timing of Surgery	**Indication**
Urgent	Cancer, severe symptoms
Elective, soon	Polyposis without obvious cancer but with symptoms
Elective, may be deferred	Age <16, asymptomatic, mild polyposis, no cancer, high desmoid risk, difficult pouch surgery

is best. Patients with severe polyposis can undergo a "staged" IPAA, first having an IRA and then a proctectomy and pouch some years later. This allows better bowel function and a less complex and less complicated surgery early on, during formative years. In patients at high risk of developing desmoid disease, surgery can also be deferred. As long as surgery is deferred, patients should have a yearly colonoscopy to make sure that the colorectal polyposis is not dangerous.

GASTRODUODENAL POLYPS

Almost all FAP patients develop gastric and duodenal polyps.[30] These are rarely problematic in patients younger than 20 years and screening endoscopy doesn't need to start until then. Gastric fundic gland polyps are non-neoplastic, hyperplastic type polyps than can be numerous but do not need to be removed. Recent reports describe a high incidence of dysplasia in random biopsies from fundic gland polyps[31] but the risk of gastric cancer in patients living in Western societies is very low. In fact, gastric cancer risk may have more to do with the gastric antral adenomas that can be found in 10% of Western FAP patients.[30] Of more importance are duodenal adenomas, found in 92% of patients with FAP. These are precursor lesions to duodenal cancer, the third most common cause of death in FAP patients behind colorectal cancer and desmoid disease.[32]

Duodenal adenomas in FAP can be staged according to the Spigelman Staging system.[33] This staging system is used to determine surveillance intervals and surgery. Recommendations are based on recent evidence that 36% of patients with Stage IV duodenal adenomatosis will develop cancer,[34] and the experience that treatment of established duodenal cancer has a poor outcome.[35]

Surveillance of the duodenum is done with both side- and end-viewing endoscopes so that easy inspection and biopsy of the duodenal ampulla can be achieved.[36] The recurrence rate of adenomas after endoscopic removal is high[37] and so no attempt is made to "clear" the duodenum[35]; however, representative biopsies are important to allow accurate staging. **Table 5** provides a suggested surveillance plan.

The surgical approach to duodenal adenomas ranges from transduodenal polypectomy, to ampullectomy, to pancreas-preserving duodenectomy (PPD), to pancreaticoduodenectomy (Whipple). For Stage IV, benign disease, PPD offers good clearance of disease, low recurrence, and low morbidity.[38] For cancer, the Whipple

Table 5	
Recommendations for duodenal surveillance in familial adenomatous polyposis	
Spigelman Stage	**Suggested Interval to Next Surveillance**
I	5 years
II	3 years
III	6 months to 1 year
IV	Strongly consider duodenectomy

procedure is the only option. Concerns that upper gastrointestinal surgery may worsen bowel function in patients who have had colectomy have not proven to be well founded. (Karlv Y, Church J, Burke C, et al. Unpublished data).

DESMOID DISEASE

After colorectal cancer, desmoid disease is the most common cause of death in patients with FAP.[32] It is an overgrowth of fibro-aponeurotic tissue related to loss of APC function and similar to sporadic desmoid tumors associated with a β catenin mutation.[39] In FAP, the desmoid disease is concentrated in the abdomen, especially in the small bowel mesentery, where its appearance ranges from flat white sheets (desmoid reaction) that pucker the mesentery and can cause kinking and obstruction of the bowel, to tumor masses that can have pressure effects on neighboring organs. About 15% of desmoid tumors in FAP grow in the abdominal wall, where they are obvious as a hard lump. A minority occur in extra-abdominal locations.

Overall, about 31% of FAP patients develop desmoid disease, 3% of which have the disease at the time of their first abdominal surgery.[40] Not all FAP patients are at equal risk of developing desmoid disease. The main risk factors are female gender,[40] genotype 3' of codon 1440,[41] a family history of desmoids,[42] and the appearance of the manifestations of Gardner's syndrome.[43] These latter factors are related. A desmoid risk factor has been reported that allows estimation of desmoid risk and the possibility of avoiding desmoid disease by deferring surgery or using sulindac as prophylaxis. Eighty percent of intra-abdominal desmoid disease occurs after abdominal surgery, and there is a hint that minimally invasive IPAA is particularly "desmoidogenic."[44]

Desmoid disease may present incidentally, during laparotomy, or may be found on a CT scan done for a different indication. This may affect surgical strategy during laparotomy in patients who have had an IRA and need proctectomy for increasing rectal polyposis. Desmoid disease in the small bowel mesentery may prevent an IPAA, or at least may make the surgery more difficult.[39,45] Patients need to be warned of this possibility. Desmoid disease also presents with symptoms, most commonly pain. This may be a result of bowel obstruction, ureteric obstruction, perforation with infection and fistula, or tumor necrosis. The best modality for imaging is with CT scan, although MRI scans avoid radiation.

There is no predictably effective treatment for desmoid disease. A staging system has been described to allow rational treatment decisions.[46,47] This is shown in **Box 1**

Suggestions for treatment of Stage I disease include nothing or sulindac, a nonsteroidal, anti-inflammatory drug that also inhibits adenoma growth. Stage II disease may be treated with sulindac with or without an estrogen blocking drug such as tamoxifen (120 mg per day) or raloxifene (120 mg per day). Patients with Stage III disease need

---

Box 1

A staging system for intra-abdominal desmoid disease in FAP

Stage I Asymptomatic disease, and not growing, and <10 cm in maximum diameter

Stage II Minimally symptomatic, and not growing, or >10 cm in maximum diameter

Stage III Symptomatic disease, or slowly growing, or obstructive complications

Stage IV Symptomatic disease, and rapidly growing, or severe complications (eg, fistula)

Data from Church J, Lynch C, Neary P, et al. A desmoid tumor-staging system separates patients with intra-abdominal, familial adenomatous polyposis-associated desmoid disease by behavior and prognosis. Dis Colon Rectum 2008;51:897–901.

chemotherapy, usually with methotrexate and vinorelbine, whereas Stage IV patients are often given adriamycin-based chemotherapy.[47–49] Several other medications have been tried, some with anecdotal success (gleevec, interferon alpha, toremifene). Surgery has been used for abdominal wall and extra-abdominal tumors with success, although recurrence rates are high. Surgery has not been encouraged for intra-abdominal desmoids because of the potential for loss of small bowel, the high morbidity, and the very high recurrence rates.[49] Recently, however, more favorable data have been reported that might encourage a more liberal use of surgery for intra-abdominal tumors. (Church J, Xhaja X, Vogel J, et al. Unpublished data).

SUMMARY

Patients with FAP are guaranteed to have one major abdominal surgery in their life. They are also subject to cancers and benign disorders in other organ systems, some of which can be life threatening. Steering a course through life while avoiding preventable disease and complications of treatment, and maintaining good quality of life is a major challenge for health care givers, patients, and their families. A successful voyage calls for good clinical cooperation between providers and patients, education and understanding, and expertise and experience. FAP patients and families need to be involved in a registry or genetic center, not to the exclusion of local practitioners but to their benefit. In this way the best of care is given and the best of outcomes ensured.

REFERENCES

1. Hernegger GS, Moore HG, Guillem JG. Attenuated familial adenomatous polyposis: an evolving and poorly understood entity. Dis Colon Rectum 2002;45:127–34.
2. Lefevre JH, Parc Y, Svrcek M, et al. APC, MYH, and the correlation genotype–phenotype in colorectal polyposis. Ann Surg Oncol 2009 [Epub ahead of print].
3. Bouquen G, Manfredi S, Blayau M, et al. Colorectal adenomatous polyposis associated with MYH mutations: genotype and phenotype characteristics. Dis Colon Rectum 2007;50:1612–7.
4. Chargelaigue A. Des polyps du rectum. Thesis, Paris, 1859.
5. Cripps WH. Two cases of disseminated polypus of the rectum. Tr Path Soc London 1882;33:165–8.
6. Bickersteth RA. Multiple polypi of the rectum occurring in a mother and child. St Barts Hosp Rep 1890;26:299–301.
7. Lockhart-Mummery JP. The causation and treatment of multiple adenomatosis of the colon. Ann Surg 1934;99:178–84.
8. Kinzler KW, Nilbert MC, Su LK, et al. Identification of FAP locus genes from chromosome-5q21. Science 1991;253:661–5.
9. Iwama T, Mishima Y, Utsunomiya J. The impact of familial adenomatous polyposis on the tumorigenesis and mortality at the several organs. Its rational treatment. Ann Surg 1993;217:101–8.
10. Park JG, Park KJ, Ahn YO, et al. Risk of gastric cancer among Korean familial adenomatous polyposis patients. Report of three cases. Dis Colon Rectum 1992;35:996–8.
11. Fearnhead NS, Britton MP, Bodmer WF. The ABC of APC. Hum Mol Genet 2001; 10:721–33.
12. van der Luijt RB, Khan PM, Vasen HF, et al. Molecular analysis of the APC gene in 105 Dutch kindreds with familial adenomatous polyposis: 67 germline mutations identified by DGGE, PTT, and southern analysis. Hum Mutat 1997;9:7–16.

13. Petersen GM. Genetic testing and counseling in familial adenomatous polyposis. Oncology (Williston Park) 1996;10:89–94.
14. Bonardi M, Bova K, LaGuardia L, et al. There is something about a new mutation that causes severe disease in FAP: a comparative study of probands stratified by family history. Dis Colon Rectum 2006;49:721–2.
15. Bülow C, Bülow S, Nielsen TF, et al. Prognosis in familial adenomatous polyposis. Results from the Polyposis Registry. Ugeskr Laeger 1996;158:4188–90.
16. Church J, Burke C, McGannon E, et al. Predicting polyposis severity by proctoscopy: how reliable is it? Dis Colon Rectum 2001;44:1249–54.
17. Church JM, Fazio VW, Lavery IC, et al. Quality of life after prophylactic colectomy and ileorectal anastomosis in patients with familial adenomatous polyposis. Dis Colon Rectum 1996;39:1404–8.
18. Aziz O, Athanasiou T, Fazio VW, et al. Meta-analysis of observational studies of ileorectal versus ileal pouch-anal anastomosis for familial adenomatous polyposis. Br J Surg 2006;93(4):407–17.
19. Olsen KO, Juul S, Bulow S, et al. Female fecundity before and after operation for familial adenomatous polyposis. Br J Surg 2003;90:227–31.
20. Remzi FH, Church JM, Bast J, et al. Mucosectomy vs. stapled ileal pouch-anal anastomosis in patients with familial adenomatous polyposis: functional outcome and neoplasia control. Dis Colon Rectum 2001;44(11):1590–6.
21. Feinberg SM, Jagelman DG, Sarre RG, et al. Spontaneous resolution of rectal polyps in patients with familial polyposis following abdominal colectomy and ileorectal anastomosis. Dis Colon Rectum 1988;31(3):169–75.
22. Lynch HT, Thorson AG, Smyrk T. Rectal cancer after prolonged sulindac chemoprevention. A case report. Cancer 1995;75(4):936–8.
23. von Roon AC, Tekkis PP, Lovegrove RE, et al. Comparison of outcomes of ileal pouch-anal anastomosis for familial adenomatous polyposis with and without previous ileorectal anastomosis. Br J Surg 2008;95(4):494–8.
24. Soravia C, O'Connor BI, Berk T, et al. Functional outcome of conversion of ileorectal anastomosis to ileal pouch-anal anastomosis in patients with familial adenomatous polyposis and ulcerative colitis. Dis Colon Rectum 1999;42(7):903–8.
25. Ziv Y, Fazio VW, Church JM, et al. Stapled ileal pouch anal anastomoses are safer than handsewn anastomoses in patients with ulcerative colitis. Am J Surg 1996;171(3):320–3.
26. Church J. Ileoanal pouch neoplasia in familial adenomatous polyposis: an underestimated threat. Dis Colon Rectum 2005;48(9):1708–13.
27. Weston-Petrides GK, Lovegrove RE, Tilney HS, et al. Comparison of outcomes after restorative proctocolectomy with or without defunctioning ileostomy. Arch Surg 2008;143:406–12.
28. Wu JS, McGannon EA, Church JM. Incidence of neoplastic polyps in the ileal pouch of patients with familial adenomatous polyposis after restorative proctocolectomy. [see comment]. Dis Colon Rectum 1998;41:552–6.
29. Church JM, McGannon E, Burke C, et al. Teenagers with familial adenomatous polyposis: what is their risk for colorectal cancer? Dis Colon Rectum 2002;45:887–9.
30. Church JM, McGannon E, Hull-Boiner, et al. Gastroduodenal polyps in patients with familial adenomatous polyposis. Dis Colon Rectum 1992;35:1170–3.
31. Bianchi LK, Burke CA, Bennett AE, et al. Fundic gland polyp dysplasia is common in familial adenomatous polyposis. Clin Gastroenterol Hepatol 2008;6:180–5.
32. Arvanitis ML, Jagelman DG, Fazio VW, et al. Mortality in patients with familial adenomatous polyposis. Dis Colon Rectum 1990;33:639–42.

33. Spigelman AD, Williams CB, Talbot IC, et al. Upper gastrointestinal cancer in patients with familial adenomatous polyposis. Lancet 1989;2(8666):783–5.

34. Groves CJ, Saunders B, Spigelman A, et al. Duodenal cancer in patients with familial adenomatous polyposis (FAP): results of a 10 year prospective study. Gut 2002;50:636–41.

35. Penna C, Bataille N, Balladur P, et al. Surgical treatment of severe duodenal polyposis in familial adenomatous polyposis. Br J Surg 1998;85:665–8.

36. Burke CA, Beck GJ, Church JM, et al. The natural history of untreated duodenal and ampullary adenomas in patients with familial adenomatous polyposis followed in an endoscopic surveillance program. Gastrointest Endosc 1999;49: 358–64.

37. Helskanen I, Kollokumpu I, Jarvinen H. Management of duodenal adenomas in 98 patients with familial adenomatous polyposis. Endoscopy 1999;31:412–6.

38. Mackey R, Walsh RM, Chung R, et al. Pancreas-sparing duodenectomy is effective management for familial adenomatous polyposis. J Gastrointest Surg 2005;9: 1088–93.

39. Kotiligam D, Lazar AJ, Pollock RE, et al. Desmoid tumor: a disease opportune for molecular insights. Histol Histopathol 2008;23:117–26.

40. Hartley JE, Church JM, Gupta S, et al. Significance of incidental desmoids identified during surgery for familial adenomatous polyposis. Dis Colon Rectum 2004; 47:334–8.

41. Nieuwenhuis MH, De Vos Tot Nederveen Cappel W, Botma A, et al. Desmoid tumors in a Dutch cohort of patients with familial adenomatous polyposis. Clin Gastroenterol Hepatol 2008;6:215–9.

42. Lefevre JH, Parc Y, Kerneis S, et al. Risk factors for development of desmoid tumours in familial adenomatous polyposis. Br J Surg 2008;95:1136–9.

43. Church J, Manilich E, LaGuardia L, et al. Can desmoids be predicted? The use of knowledge discovery techniques in familial adenomatous polyposis. Dis Colon Rectum 2006;49:722.

44. Vogel J, Church JM, LaGuardia L. Minimally invasive pouch surgery predisposes to desmoid tumor formation in patients with familial adenomatous polyposis. Dis Colon Rectum 2005;48:662–3.

45. Penna C, Tiret E, Parc R, et al. Operation and abdominal desmoid tumors in familial adenomatous polyposis. Surg Gynecol Obstet 1993;177:263–8.

46. Church J, Lynch C, Neary P, et al. A desmoid tumor-staging system separates patients with intra-abdominal, familial adenomatous polyposis-associated desmoid disease by behavior and prognosis. Dis Colon Rectum 2008;51:897–901.

47. Church J, Berk T, Boman BM, et al. Collaborative Group of the Americas on Inherited Colorectal Cancer. Staging intra-abdominal desmoid tumors in familial adenomatous polyposis: a search for a uniform approach to a troubling disease. Dis Colon Rectum 2005;48:1528–34.

48. Okuno S. The enigma of desmoid tumors. Curr Treat Opt Oncol 2006;7:438–43.

49. Sturt NJ, Clark SK. Current ideas in desmoid tumours. Fam Cancer 2006;5: 275–85.

MUTYH-Associated Polyposis and Colorectal Cancer

Malcolm G. Dunlop, MD*, Susan M. Farrington, PhD

KEYWORDS

- Colorectal cancer • Polyposis • Genetic • Susceptibility
- Base excision repair • MUTYH

The autosomal dominant disorders (genes responsible in parentheses), Lynch syndrome (DNA mismatch repair genes), familial adenomatous polyposis, or FAP (APC), Peutz-Jeghers syndrome (LKB1), and juvenile polyposis (SMAD4, BMPR1A), are associated with a high risk of colorectal cancer for relatives of affected cases. Although penetrance is high, these syndromes constitute only a minority of the excess familial risk of colorectal cancer because of the low frequency of pathogenic alleles in the general population.[1] In contrast, evidence from family studies in which study subjects have been categorized by molecular analysis for high-penetrance alleles indicate that much of the residual excess risk outside these disorders is consistent with other modes of inheritance.[2–4] Several common low-penetrance variants have already been shown to contribute to the residual risk component, consistent with a polygenic model of colorectal cancer susceptibility.[5] High-penetrance, recessive alleles, however, also make up part of that excess risk.

Inactivating variants in the base excision repair (BER) gene, MUTYH, have been shown to account for up to 50% of APC mutation–negative polyposis cases[6] and 0.2% to 0.9% of all colorectal cancer cases, with a recessive mode of inheritance associated with a high cancer risk. The population frequency of common alleles in caucasian populations (>80% of all proved pathogenic mutations) is approximately 0.2%,[4,7,8] and this is reflected in a low homozygote frequency (approximately 1/10,000) in control populations.[4,7] This article reviews the role of defective BER, and MUTYH specifically, in colorectal cancer etiology and discusses the consequences of MUTYH gene defects, with particular emphasis on clinical relevance to colorectal polyposis, colorectal cancer risk, and appraising the risk of extracolonic

Relevant work in the authors' laboratory is supported by the Scottish Government Chief Scientist's Office (CZB/4/449), Cancer Research UK (C348/A8896, C48/A6361), and a centre grant from CORE Charity as part of the Digestive Cancer Campaign.
Colon Cancer Genetics Group, Institute of Genetics and Molecular Medicine, University of Edinburgh and MRC Human Genetics Unit, Western General Hospital, Edinburgh EH4 2XU, UK
* Corresponding author.
E-mail address: malcolm.dunlop@hgu.mrc.ac.uk (M.G. Dunlop).

Surg Oncol Clin N Am 18 (2009) 599–610
doi:10.1016/j.soc.2009.08.003
1055-3207/09/$ – see front matter © 2009 Elsevier Inc. All rights reserved.

malignancy. Evidence guiding clinical practice, in terms of surveillance recommendations and the options for surgical and other prophylactic interventions, is reviewed.

IDENTIFICATION OF MUTYH AS A SUSCEPTIBILITY GENE FOR COLORECTAL NEOPLASIA

In 2002, Al-Tassan and colleagues[9,10] reported a study in which they characterized somatic mutations in the APC gene within polyps arising in a polyposis family with three affected members, all of whom were negative for germline mutations in the APC gene. They observed an excess of somatic G:T transversion mutations in the APC gene and, recognizing such mutations as the hallmark of oxidative DNA damage, they investigated the possibility that these were a manifestation of a constitutional defect in BER. This proved to be the case, and missense germline mutations (Y179C and G396D) were identified in the BER gene, MUTYH, in affected family members. Y179C and G396D have proved the most common in caucasian populations and functional assays of adenine glycosylase activity of both mutant proteins demonstrated significantly reduced function, especially for the Y179C variant, establishing that inactivation of both alleles of MUTYH is associated with a polyposis syndrome.[9,10] The MUTYH gene maps to chromosomal region 1p34.3-p32.1 and encodes a 535 amino acid protein, which functions as a glycosylase and participates in the BER pathway. Mutations identified by Al-Tassan and colleagues were at highly conserved residues. The Y179C mutation affects MUTYH mismatch specificity, whereas G396D seems to affect substrate binding.

Segregation in the original family[9] was consistent with recessive inheritance and this was confirmed in a larger set of polyposis families that were negative for germline APC mutations.[11] Subsequent studies of larger groups of polyposis patients confirmed the observation and have further refined understanding about the mode of inheritance and the phenotypic associations.[6,12-14]

It is now standard clinical genetics practice to undertake MUTYH mutation analysis in all APC-negative polyposis cases, emphasizing the clinical impact of the original observations. Although some of the polyposis patients studied to date have concurrent colorectal cancer, such cases are highly selected and likely the subject of ascertainment bias, falsely elevating the risk of colorectal cancer. Hence, it was not definitively established whether or not MUTYH mutations also predisposed to colorectal cancer. Case-control studies, however, confirmed the association between biallelic MUTYH mutations and colorectal cancer risk,[15-18] subsequently extended to larger sample sets.[4,7,8]

The protein product of MUTYH is one of several participants in the BER pathway that identifies and repairs oxidative damage of DNA (discussed later). Several studies have analyzed the genes encoding two other key components (OGG1, MTH1) of that pathway, but mutations in these genes have not been linked convincingly with colorectal polyposis or with colorectal cancer.[19] Thus, there is no current evidence of locus heterogeneity for BER-related polyposis and, for practical purposes, inactivating germline mutations in MUTYH can be considered as the sole defective BER gene linked with colorectal cancer risk.

OUTLINE OF BASE EXCISION REPAIR AND RELEVANCE TO COLORECTAL NEOPLASIA

Reactive oxygen species (ROS), including hydrogen peroxide, superoxide, and hydroxyl radicals, are generated as byproducts of aerobic cellular metabolism and are toxic to DNA. ROS are also produced as part of the inflammatory response and as a consequence of environmental stresses. Nucleotide bases, especially guanine, are highly sensitive to oxidative damage. 8-oxo-7, 8-dihydro2'deoxyguanosine (8-oxo-G) is a stable and highly mutagenic product of oxidative DNA damage, prone to postreplicative mispairings of 8-oxo-G:A, G:A, or C:A.[20] The mechanism of BER in removing oxidative damage involves a series of sequential steps requiring component proteins and complex interactions with other repair pathways and the DNA replication machinery.

BER is highly conserved throughout evolution because of its pivotal importance in maintaining genomic stability. The main function of MUTYH, inferred from its *Escherichia coli* homolog, MutY, is recognition and removal of adenine bases from 8-oxo-G:A, G:A, or C:A mispairs. DNA mismatch repair is also activated by oxidative DNA damage via the MutSα complex,[21] whereas MUTYH also interacts directly with MSH6 protein.[22] DNA mismatch repair proteins may also play a role in removing oxidative lesions from the nucleotide pool itself.[23]

MUTYH has a high degree of substrate specificity for GAA, a sequence that has a particular predilection for G:C>T:A transversion mutations, resulting in a STOP codon (TAA) in the APC gene itself. The many GAA sequences in the APC gene, and the fact that the large bowel epithelium is exposed to high levels of ROS through diet and inflammatory mediators, may explain why colorectal neoplasms are a particular feature of defective BER. Despite the importance in BER function of the glycosylase, OGG1, and the nucleoside triphosphatase, MTH1, there is no convincing evidence to link mutations in these genes, or any other components of the BER pathway, with colorectal cancer.[19] Similarly, despite anecdotal reports of MUTYH defects in association with lung, breast, gastric, and endometrial cancer, there is no definitive evidence for an elevated risk of such cancers.

MOLECULAR PATHOGENESIS OF COLORECTAL NEOPLASIA IN MUTYH-ASSOCIATED POLYPOSIS

Understanding how BER defects influence tumor initiation and progression in colorectal epithelial cells is of considerable biologic and clinical interest. The initial identification of MUTYH defects and the resultant transversion mutations in the APC gene gave some mechanistic clue as to how MUTYH null cells may influence tumor formation.[24]

As discussed previously, G:C>T:A transversion mutations are a hallmark of defective BER. This can result in truncating mutations in the APC gene in colonic epithelial cells. Similarly, another gene frequently mutated in colorectal tumors, the proto-oncogene, K-Ras, has been shown to have an excess of transversion mutations in biallelic MUTYH carriers. The K-Ras mutation spectrum is more restricted than that in APC, because most reported mutations comprise a G>C transversion at codon 12, G12C.[25,26] Thus, defective BER effectively foreshortens the timeline of mutation accumulation in key genes involved in colorectal carcinogensis through failure to control the normal rate of mutation. It may be suspected that mutations in other genes could also be observed in BER defective cases but to date none have been apparent other than APC and K-Ras.

MUTYH ALLELES ARE INHERITED AS A RECESSIVE TRAIT

Segregation studies indicate that MUTYH-associated colorectal polyposis and colorectal cancers arising in such cases are inherited as a recessive trait.[9,11] This has implications for counseling families (see articles elsewhere in this issue by Aronson and Hempel) and for clinical surveillance. Some studies have reported segregation as an apparently dominant mode of inheritance in approximately 15% to 30% of families (reviewed by Poulsen and Bisgaard),[12] but the overwhelming weight of evidence from large population-based studies indicates that MUTYH-associated colorectal neoplasia is inherited as a recessive trait.[4,6–8,17] Nevertheless, it is important to understand the clinical relevance of factors that underlie pseudodominant inheritance. Apparent dominant inheritance in a family with an individual carrying biallelic MUTYH mutations may be due to confounding factors, such as cosegregation of another polyposis gene or a high-penetrance cancer gene (eg, APC or DNA mismatch repair gene), ascertainment bias, unassociated cancer cases (phenocopies), and even rare instances of biallelic cases in prior generations. Thus, pedigree tracing is essential to document family history from all individuals with biallelic MUTYH mutations who have polyposis or colorectal cancer. In particular, FAP and Lynch syndrome should always be considered, if only to be excluded, and this is usually best achieved through referral for formal clinical genetics management.

COLORECTAL CANCER RISK ASSOCIATED WITH HETEROZYGOUS MUTYH ALLELES

There remains ongoing controversy regarding whether or not there is a marginally increased risk of colorectal cancer in heterozygote carriers of MUTYH alleles.[4,7,15,17,27,28] Several large studies have revisited this issue, reporting a significantly elevated risk to the monoallelic carriers (genotype relative risk [GRR] 1.28[8] and age-adjusted odds ratio 1.48[7]) contrasting with another recent large study where no effect was observed (GRR 1.07, not significant) in the primary data or in a meta-analysis of published data available to that date.[4] Supporting the notion that heterozygous mutations may not be associated with an elevated risk, animal studies have shown that monoallelic inactivation of MUTYH does not result in a demonstrable increase in tumor burden in a Min mouse background nor is there any change in the proportion of somatic *APC* G:T transversion mutations.[29] It is conceivable that the excess risk to monoallelic carriers observed in population studies[7,8] could be due to unidentified compound heterozygotes, for MUTYH or other BER gene alleles, but this seems unlikely because resequencing of MUTYH has generally been performed and there is little evidence of pathogenic mutations in other BER genes.[8]

To some extent, the argument about a monoallelic MUTYH effect may bemuse clinicians, because it may seem only of academic and biologic interest. There are practical clinical implications, however, because when a biallelic carrier is identified, monoallelic carriers are identified in offspring, parents, and siblings. The risk to heterozygotes is modest, even at the most extreme of available estimates (OR 1.5), so carriers should be counseled accordingly. It is not appropriate to offer more intensive screening than that of the general population. Nonetheless, the potential excess risk to heterozygotes may have public health implications if genetic risk stratification were introduced for the whole population. For the present, population screening for BER gene alleles is impractical because of allelic heterogeneity and also because of the low frequency of any of the alleles. Hence, the implications are largely clinical genetic to reassure relatives in the process of family counseling.

In summary, it remains somewhat controversial whether or not there is an excess risk to monoallelic carriers who are relatives of index biallelic carriers, despite the large numbers of subjects in the available studies. Even at the extreme of the available estimates, however, that risk is not sufficiently high to merit recommending surveillance over and above that for average-risk individuals in the general population.

CLINICAL GENETICS ISSUES FOR RELATIVES OF AN INDEX BIALLELIC CARRIER CASE

Although this scenario may change in the future, if MUTYH mutation analysis was widened to include all cancer cases and even the general population, currently the most common way in which biallelic carriers are identified is through diagnosis of multiple polyposis with, or without, an established colorectal cancer in a patient with a negative APC mutation test. In some instances, family history may already indicate a recessive mode of inheritance, with one or more siblings affected and parents unaffected. Rarely, families may exhibit pseudodominant segregation. In all circumstances, it is important that APC mutations have been excluded in the index case of polyposis. The issue of cancer risk to the immediate family should be discussed and the family offered genetic counseling through contact by the proband. Because the disorder is fully recessive, the prior risk is 25% of biallelic carrier status in siblings.

A variety of mutations in MUTYH have been reported, with the largest study of polyposis families reporting 36 different mutations in 185 patients of European extraction.[6] The missense mutations, Y179C and G396D, represented 44% and 24% of all mutations respectively, whereas truncating mutations were identified in another 17%. Although many previous studies have restricted analysis to the common variants (Y179C and G396D), the mutation spectrum reported in this large study emphasizes the need to analyze the entire MUTYH gene to fully explore the role of MUTYH in polyposis and colorectal cancer.

Given the high penetrance for cancer, MUTYH mutation analysis should be offered to all siblings. Parents and offspring are unlikely to be at greatly elevated risk because they likely carry only one pathogenic allele, notwithstanding the contentious marginal elevation in heterozygote risk. Where possible, however, both parents of the index case should be tested to exclude the rare possibility that one is a nonpenetrant biallelic carrier. Furthermore, the other parent of any offspring from the proband should also be tested for at least the common MUTYH alleles (approximately 2% allele frequency) and children tested only if relevant. These simple and inexpensive measures would essentially rule out the possibility of inappropriate reassurance during family counseling. The objective is to identify biallelic carriers in the family context to instigate appropriate clinical surveillance and discuss prophylactic surgery (discussed later). If genetic testing is declined by particular family members for personal or health insurance reasons, however, then a recommendation for colonoscopic surveillance should be made to siblings but not to offspring or parents, other than routine average-risk screening.

PATHOLOGY AND TUMOR MICROSATELLITE INSTABILITY STATUS

Several studies have addressed the pathologic features of MUTYH-associated large bowel neoplasia and found no pathognomonic features associated with biallelic MUTYH mutations.[7,30] Polyps can be exclusively adenomatous or mixed adenomatous and hyperplastic. Cancer arising in MUTYH carriers is distributed throughout the length of the large bowel, and there is an excess of proximal cancers compared with the generality of colorectal cancer, where distal tumors are more common.[4,7] There are no characteristic histopathology or clinicopathogic features that distinguish MUTYH-associated carcinomas.[4,6,7,30] Although MUTYH-associated polyposis tends to comprise an attenuated phenotype, with fewer polyps than in FAP and a preponderance of proximal colonic cancer, none of these features has particularly good discriminatory value in identifying mutation carriers. The relationship with microsatellite instability is one of almost mutual exclusivity.[4,7,18,26] Because most sporadic colorectal cancers are microsatellite stable in any case, however, microsatellite instability is not a particularly useful predictor of the presence of MUTYH mutations.[4]

Biallelic MUTYH mutations are variously reported in the range of 26% to 50% for patients with 10 to 100 polyps and 7% to 29% for patients with 100 to 1000 polyps.[6] In contrast, biallelic mutations are rare in patients with fewer than 10 adenomas included in registry-based studies of APC-negative polyposis families.[6,31] Of biallelic carriers in population-based studies of colorectal cancer, 20% to 50% have no current or past history of associated polyps.[4,7,17]

Taking into account practical considerations, it seems reasonable to consider referral for genetic counseling and mutation analysis of the MUTYH gene for all patients with a cumulative load of 10 or more adenomas, with or without colorectal cancer. This will not identify all MUTYH carriers, but currently it is not feasible to screen MUTYH for mutations in the general population or even in all cases of colorectal cancer outside of research projects. Thus, in clinical practice, most index biallelic carriers will continue to be identified through polyposis cases in which the APC gene has been shown to be free of mutations or colorectal cancer cases of concurrent or a past history of multiple polyps.

POPULATION DIFFERENCES IN ALLELE FREQUENCY

Because MUTYH polyposis has only recently been characterized at the molecular level and allele frequency in the general population is low, studies in the literature from various populations comprise relatively small numbers of subjects. Furthermore, most biallelic carriers identified to date were selected on polyposis or cancer phenotype, so differential ascertainment bias between the various reported populations may confound comparisons of allele frequency in affected cases. The mutation frequency in MUTYH and the relative contributions of the two most common variants has been reviewed.[12] Although Y179C and G396D seem more common in caucasian than in Asian populations, the data are too limited outside of populations of European extraction to place much emphasis on population differences at this stage, given the small number of subjects studied.

AGE AT ONSET OF COLORECTAL POLYPOSIS AND CANCER

In the absence of sufficiently large numbers of documented biallelic mutations carriers with prospective follow-up, estimation of penetrance is necessarily indirect. Furthermore, colorectal neoplasia is common in the general population, so phenocopies can arise. Notwithstanding these methodologic problems and the likely overestimation of risk, analysis of age at polyposis onset reveals that essentially all biallelic carriers have developed multiple polyps by age 65.[6] The Y179C MUTYH allele is associated with a more severe phenotype than G396D, because polyposis has earlier onset and the cancer risk is higher. The severe phenotype associated with Y179C has also been observed in a large case-control study of colorectal cancer, manifesting as an earlier age of onset and an greater overall risk associated with the Y179C allele.[4] These clinical observations are supported by laboratory studies that show that Y179C results in a lower MUTYH expression than does G396D[9,32] and also has an impact on 8-oxo-G:A mismatch recognition to a greater extent than does the G396D variant. Thus, there do seem to be genotype-phenotype correlations in MUTYH-associated colorectal neoplasia, at least for the two common alleles in European populations. Genotype information may help guide decision making on surveillance and on prophylactic surgery (discussed later).

CLINICAL SURVEILLANCE OF THE LARGE BOWEL FOR BIALLELIC MUTYH CARRIERS

There have been no prospective studies examining the effectiveness of colonosopic surveillance and polypectomy in preventing colorectal cancer or cancer-related mortality in biallelic MUTYH carriers. Much of the available indirect evidence is from descriptive studies, so benefit has yet to be definitively established. Nonetheless, the overall lifetime risk of colorectal cancer is high[4,7,8,17] and risk is strongly age dependent, with the highest risk in younger age groups.[4] Because the evidence from FAP and attenuated FAP is so compelling, surveillance is now considered the standard of care in MUTYH-associated neoplasia.[33] The mean age of cancer onset in unselected cancer cases is 47 years. The distribution of age at onset for cancer, however, is best estimated from population-based studies.[4,7,8,15,17] The relatively small numbers of biallelic carriers, even in these large studies, mean that the confidence intervals are wide. Approximately 75% of biallelic carriers have developed colorectal cancer by age 60, and, for practical purposes, the cumulative cancer risk can be assumed to be approximately 50% by age 50, 66% by age 60, and over 80% by age 70. Over and above cancer detection, there is value in identifying carriers with an adenoma load. Cancer-free or polyposis-free control subjects with biallelic MUTYH mutations reported in the literature are exceptionally rare. Only two control subjects with biallelic mutations have ever been reported, one of whom was shown to have polyposis on colonoscopy[7] and the other is less than 60 years old.[4] Expert opinion based on a synthesis of available evidence at the time has suggested that surveillance should start between the ages of 18 and 20.[33] Commencing surveillance at age 25, however, also is reasonable given the lack of any reported cancer cases before that age. Colonoscopy is the preferred surveillance modality because polyps and cancers arise throughout the length of the bowel, with an excess proportion in the proximal colon.[4] The screening interval should be 2 to 3 yearly, somewhat less intensive than that recommended for attenuated FAP.[33] Again, however, these screening intervals are not well grounded in evidence base. As discussed previously, those with monoallelic MUTYH mutations have only marginally increased cancer risk, so aggressive colonoscopic surveillance is unnecessary.

EXTRACOLONIC FEATURES AND SURVEILLANCE

Gastroduodenal polyposis has been observed in approximately 20% of MUTYH biallelic carriers[34,35] but most of these studies were from highly selected polyposis registry families, so this is likely an overestimate. Nonetheless, 3- to 5-year upper gastrointestinal (GI) surveillance is recommended from age 30 and this should be with forward and side-viewing endoscopes to fully inspect the duodenal ampulla. The evidence for benefit in MUTYH-associated polyposis (MAP) is indirect and even less compelling than for FAP. This approach, however, seems reasonable, given several reports of upper GI cancer arising in biallelic carriers.[13,34–36] Similarly, FAP-associated extraintestinal features, such as osteomas and congenital hypertrophy of the retinal pigment epithelium, have been reported only anecdotally in MUTYH biallelic carriers. Overall, the risk is heavily biased toward the large bowel and there is no compelling evidence to support any other form of surveillance. The tentative evidence of upper GI cancer and the ready screening access mean that upper GI surveillance is reasonable.

OPPORTUNISTIC SURGICAL PROPHYLAXIS FOR BIALLELIC MUTYH MUTATION CARRIERS WITH ESTABLISHED COLORECTAL CANCER OR POLYPOSIS NOT AMENABLE TO ENDOSCOPIC MANAGEMENT

Consider a scenario where a patient with cancer or polyposis who requires a colorectal resection is already known to be biallelic carrier during preoperative work-up. The availability of information on MUTYH mutation status to inform surgical decision making will become more commonplace as biallelic carriers are entered into surveillance programs. Cases will become apparent due to the presence of cancer at initial colonoscopy, the development of an interval cancer, or the presence of multiple polyps that are not amenable to endoscopic resection.

Surgical strategy for the colon or rectum will partly be determined by the location of the tumor, given the preponderance of more proximal tumors. Furthermore, there is a propensity for synchronous cancers in biallelic carriers, along with the likely concurrent multiple polyposis.[4,6–8,15,17,37] Hence, there is likely to be a requirement for more extensive surgery than resection of the relevant segment harboring the incident cancer itself. In addition, the requirement for surgery provides an opportunity for opportunistic prophylaxis, comprising resection of the majority or all of the at-risk large bowel epithelium to minimize future cancer risk and facilitate surveillance.

The benefit in reducing future cancer risk with only a marginal increase in morbidity means that colonic cancer is best treated by a colectomy and ileorectal anastomosis rather than a segmental resection. Restorative proctocolectomy with ileoanal pouch reconstruction is also an option, especially if many concurrent rectal polyps are a feature. For patients presenting with rectal cancer where preoperative staging indicates that cure is likely, there is considerable rationale for proctocolectomy and pouch reconstruction, because the proximal cancer risk would not be addressed by anterior resection. There is limited indirect evidence to guide surgical practice. Nonetheless, taking descriptive data on risk into account and the fact that an operation is an absolute requirement in such cases, these approaches are readily justifiable.

PROPHYLAXIS FOR BIALLELIC MUTYH MUTATION CARRIERS WITHOUT CANCER

The issues surrounding surgical resection with purely prophylactic intent are less straightforward than for patients with established cancer, because surgery would otherwise not be indicated in asymptomatic individuals. In most cases, polyp counts are low, so many cases can be controlled by endoscopic polyp removal. Prophylactic resection, however, is already becoming a clinical reality as patients are counseled about the high lifetime risk of colorectal cancer and the requirement for repeated colonoscopy over their lifetime. In one large study, 200 of 275 polyposis patients with clinical data had already had a colectomy by the time of clinical genetics referral, 68% were symptomatic, and 58% already had colorectal cancer.[6] There are no formal guidelines, however, so practice is evolving. One school of thought advocates mainly surveillance,[33] but there is also a more proactive school advocating preemptive resection.[38] In light of the documented penetrance for cancer,[4,6–8,17,38] it is clear that well-informed counseling should include consideration about prophylactic colorectal resection. Cancer history in other siblings may be helpful. Hence, the risk may be sufficiently high to merit considering prophylactic colectomy and ileorectal anastomosis or proctocolectomy and ileoanal pouch if dense rectal polyposis is a feature. The nature of the MUTYH mutation also may have an impact on decision making. Y179C is increasingly recognized as a more severe allele than G396D, because Y179C homozygotes are shown to have an earlier age of polyposis and cancer onset than G396D/Y179C compound heterozygotes or G396D/G396D homozygotes.[4,6] In summary, patients should be counseled that the cancer risk is high but there is limited available evidence to guide decisions on the effectiveness and balance of benefit for surveillance or for prophylactic surgery.

In contrast to Lynch syndrome where gynecologic cancer risk is high, so incidental prophylactic surgery could be considered in such circumstances, the lack of evidence for an excess risk of other intra-abdominal cancers means that opportunistic prophylactic removal of other organs is not appropriate when undertaking resectional surgery for MUTYH-associated colorectal neoplasia.

There is the possibility that aspirin and other chemopreventative agents may have a role in the management of MUTYH-related colorectal cancer. There is compelling evidence from observational studies and randomized trials of a risk reduction using aspirin in average-risk subjects.[39] In addition, there is some evidence that survival after cancer development is also improved.[40] Although interim analysis of the effect of aspirin on incidence reduction in mutation carriers from Lynch syndrome families did not show any benefit,[41] subsequent analysis of longer follow-up data has been presented and is encouraging. [42] Hence, there may be a place for aspirin chemoprevention in MUTYH biallelic carriers, although randomized trials to test the effect seem unlikely given the numbers of mutation carriers identified to date and the frequent requirement for preemptive resection.

SUMMARY

Defects in MUTYH seem to be the main, if not the only, genetic defects responsible for defective BER in the colorectal epithelium. Biallelic germline MUTYH mutations are associated with a high risk of polyposis and of colorectal cancer. The missense variants, Y179C and G396D, make up the majority of all mutations in polyposis cases and in colorectal cancer. With recent detailed sequence analysis, the spectrum of pathogenic mutations in MUTYH has broadened. Within the constraints of available evidence, it seems that defective BER is the key functional deficit, resulting in a failure to repair G:C>T:A transversion mutations that arise in the colonic epithelial cells as a consequence of oxidative DNA damage. The resultant mutations in APC and in K-Ras are selected for because of the key roles for these genes in colorectal carcinogenesis. Y179C has been shown convincingly to be a more severe allele than G396D, associated with earlier-onset polyposis and a greater colorectal cancer risk. Nonetheless, this is only relative to Y179C, and the risk to G396D homozygote carriers compared with average-risk populations is still high (Y179C/Y179C, GRR 57 versus G396D/G396D, GRR 20).

Multiple polyposis and colorectal cancer predisposition are common to familial APC and MUTYH-related disease. Screening for APC mutations and for (at least) the common MUTYH mutations is now standard practice in many health care systems. Colonoscopic surveillance is essential from approximately 25 years of age; some investigators suggest 18 years. As experience grows, management will evolve but the degree of colorectal cancer, the problem of symptomatic polyposis, and a requirement for lifelong colonoscopic surveillance means that it seems likely that many patients and their clinicians will opt for prophylactic surgery to control the colorectal cancer risk.

ACKNOWLEDGMENTS

The authors thank all those in the Colon Cancer Genetics Group, especially Albert Tenesa, Harry Campbell, and Evi Theodoratou, who have been pivotal to our work in the field; all those who worked on the COGS and SOCCS studies including the research nurse teams and the administrative teams; and all contributing clinicians at collaborating centers throughout Scotland.

REFERENCES

1. Dunlop MG, Farrington SM, Nicholl I, et al. Population carrier frequency of hMSH2 and hMLH1 mutations. Br J Cancer 2000;83(12):1643–5.

2. Aaltonen L, Johns L, Jarvinen H, et al. Explaining the familial colorectal cancer risk associated with mismatch repair (MMR)-deficient and MMR-stable tumors. Clin Cancer Res 2007;13(1):356–61.
3. Jenkins MA, Baglietto L, Dite GS, et al. After hMSH2 and hMLH1—what next? Analysis of three-generational, population-based, early-onset colorectal cancer families. Int J Cancer 2002;102(2):166–71.
4. Lubbe SJ, Di Bernardo MC, Chandler IP, et al. Clinical implications of the colorectal cancer risk associated with MUTYH mutation. J Clin Oncol 2009;27(24): 3975–80.
5. Tenesa A, Dunlop MG. New insights into the aetiology of colorectal cancer from genome-wide association studies. Nat Rev Genet May 12, 2009 [Epub ahead of print].
6. Nielsen M, Joerink-van de Beld MC, Jones N, et al. Analysis of MUTYH genotypes and colorectal phenotypes in patients with MUTYH-associated polyposis. Gastroenterology 2009;136(2):471–6.
7. Cleary SP, Cotterchio M, Jenkins MA, et al. Germline MutY human homologue mutations and colorectal cancer: a multisite case-control study. Gastroenterology 2009;136(4):1251–60.
8. Tenesa A, Campbell H, Barnetson R, et al. Association of MUTYH and colorectal cancer. Br J Cancer 2006;95(2):239–42.
9. Al-Tassan N, Chmiel NH, Maynard J, et al. Inherited variants of MYH associated with somatic G:C–>T:A mutations in colorectal tumors. Nat Genet 2002;30(2):227–32.
10. Jones S, Emmerson P, Maynard J, et al. Biallelic germline mutations in MYH predispose to multiple colorectal adenoma and somatic G:C–>T:A mutations. Hum Mol Genet 2002;11(23):2961–7.
11. Sampson JR, Dolwani S, Jones S, et al. Autosomal recessive colorectal adenomatous polyposis due to inherited mutations of MYH. Lancet 2003;362(9377): 39–41.
12. Poulsen ML, Bisgaard ML. MUTYH Associated Polyposis (MAP). Curr Genomics 2008;9(6):420–35.
13. Sieber OM, Lipton L, Crabtree M, et al. Multiple colorectal adenomas, classic adenomatous polyposis, and germ-line mutations in MYH. N Engl J Med 2003; 348(9):791–9.
14. Venesio T, Molatore S, Cattaneo F, et al. High frequency of MYH gene mutations in a subset of patients with familial adenomatous polyposis. Gastroenterology 2004; 126(7):1681–5.
15. Croitoru ME, Cleary SP, Di Nicola N, et al. Association between biallelic and monoallelic germline MYH gene mutations and colorectal cancer risk. J Natl Cancer Inst 2004;96(21):1631–4.
16. Enholm S, Hienonen T, Suomalainen A, et al. Proportion and phenotype of MYH-associated colorectal neoplasia in a population-based series of Finnish colorectal cancer patients. Am J Pathol 2003;163(3):827–32.
17. Farrington SM, Tenesa A, Barnetson R, et al. Germline susceptibility to colorectal cancer due to base-excision repair gene defects. Am J Hum Genet 2005;77(1): 112–9.
18. Wang L, Baudhuin LM, Boardman LA, et al. MYH mutations in patients with attenuated and classic polyposis and with young-onset colorectal cancer without polyps. Gastroenterology 2004;127(1):9–16.
19. Dallosso AR, Dolwani S, Jones N, et al. Inherited predisposition to colorectal adenomas caused by multiple rare alleles of MUTYH but not OGG1, NUDT1, NTH1 or NEIL 1, 2 or 3. Gut 2008;57(9):1252–5.

20. David SS, O'Shea VL, Kundu S. Base-excision repair of oxidative DNA damage. Nature 2007;447(7147):941–50.
21. Mazurek A, Berardini M, Fishel R. Activation of human MutS homologs by 8-oxo-guanine DNA damage. J Biol Chem 2002;277(10):8260–6.
22. Gu Y, Parker A, Wilson TM, et al. Human MutY homolog, a DNA glycosylase involved in base excision repair, physically and functionally interacts with mismatch repair proteins human MutS homolog 2/human MutS homolog 6. J Biol Chem 2002;277(13):11135–42.
23. Colussi C, Parlanti E, Degan P, et al. The mammalian mismatch repair pathway removes DNA 8-oxodGMP incorporated from the oxidized dNTP pool. Curr Biol 2002;12(11):912–8.
24. Cheadle JP, Sampson JR. MUTYH-associated polyposis–from defect in base excision repair to clinical genetic testing. DNA Repair (Amst) 2007;6(3): 274–9.
25. Kambara T, Whitehall VL, Spring KJ, et al. Role of inherited defects of MYH in the development of sporadic colorectal cancer. Genes Chromosomes Cancer 2004; 40(1):1–9.
26. Lipton L, Halford SE, Johnson V, et al. Carcinogenesis in MYH-associated poly-posis follows a distinct genetic pathway. Cancer Res 2003;63(22):7595–9.
27. Jenkins MA, Croitoru ME, Monga N, et al. Risk of colorectal cancer in monoallelic and biallelic carriers of MYH mutations: a population-based case-family study. Cancer Epidemiol Biomarkers Prev 2006;15(2):312–4.
28. Jones N, Vogt S, Nielsen M, et al. Increased colorectal cancer incidence in obli-gate carriers of heterozygous mutations in MUTYH. Gastroenterology 2009; 137(2):489–94, 494.e1; quiz 725–486.
29. Sieber OM, Howarth KM, Thirlwell C, et al. Myh deficiency enhances intestinal tumorigenesis in multiple intestinal neoplasia (ApcMin/+) mice. Cancer Res 2004;64(24):8876–81.
30. O'Shea AM, Cleary SP, Croitoru MA, et al. Pathological features of colorectal carcinomas in MYH-associated polyposis. Histopathology 2008;53(2):184–94.
31. Gismondi V, Meta M, Bonelli L, et al. Prevalence of the Y165C, G382D and 1395delGGA germline mutations of the MYH gene in Italian patients with adenomatous polyposis coli and colorectal adenomas. Int J Cancer 2004; 109(5):680–4.
32. Parker AR, Sieber OM, Shi C, et al. Cells with pathogenic biallelic mutations in the human MUTYH gene are defective in DNA damage binding and repair. Carcino-genesis 2005;26(11):2010–8.
33. Vasen HF, Moslein G, Alonso A, et al. Guidelines for the clinical management of familial adenomatous polyposis (FAP). Gut 2008;57(5):704–13.
34. Aretz S, Uhlhaas S, Goergens H, et al. MUTYH-associated polyposis: 70 of 71 patients with biallelic mutations present with an attenuated or atypical phenotype. Int J Cancer 2006;119(4):807–14.
35. Nielsen M, Poley JW, Verhoef S, et al. Duodenal carcinoma in MUTYH-associated polyposis. J Clin Pathol 2006;59(11):1212–5.
36. de Ferro SM, Suspiro A, Fidalgo P, et al. Aggressive phenotype of MYH-associ-ated polyposis with jejunal cancer and intra-abdominal desmoid tumor: report of a case. Dis Colon Rectum 2009;52(4):742–5.
37. Dolwani S, Williams GT, West KP, et al. Analysis of inherited MYH/(MutYH) muta-tions in British Asian patients with colorectal cancer. Gut 2007;56(4):593.
38. Leite JS, Isidro G, Martins M, et al. Is prophylactic colectomy indicated in patients with MYH-associated polyposis? Colorectal Dis 2005;7(4):327–31.

39. Dube C, Rostom A, Lewin G, et al. The use of aspirin for primary prevention of colorectal cancer: a systematic review prepared for the U.S. Preventive Services Task Force. Ann Intern Med 2007;146(5):365–75.

40. Chan AT, Ogino S, Fuchs CS. Aspirin use and survival after diagnosis of colorectal cancer. JAMA 2009;302(6):649–58.

41. Burn J, Bishop DT, Mecklin JP, et al. Effect of aspirin or resistant starch on colorectal neoplasia in the Lynch syndrome. N Engl J Med 2008;359(24): 2567–78.

42. Burn J. Presented at 3rd Biennial Scientific Meeting; InSiGHT conference. Dusseldorf, June, 2009. Family Cancer, in press.

The *hMSH2* and *hMLH1* Genes in Hereditary Nonpolyposis Colorectal Cancer

Patrick M. Lynch, JD, MD

KEYWORDS

- *hMSH2* gene • *hMLH1* gene • Mismatch repair genes
- Hereditary nonpolyposis colon cancer • HNPCC
- Lynch syndrome

Hereditary nonpolyposis colorectal cancer (HNPCC) is the most common inherited colorectal cancer predisposing condition. Unlike familial adenomatous polyposis (FAP) or Peutz-Jeghers (P-J) syndrome, there is no clearly diagnostic presenting feature in any given patient. The tendency toward early age at onset, multiplicity of tumors, right-sided colon involvement, characteristic tumor pathology, and spectrum of extracolonic tumors may or may not be evident. One or more such signs will often be seen in one or more relatives if details of family history can be collected. HNPCC is an important problem for the surgeon because up to 60% of carriers of mismatch repair (MMR) gene mutations develop colorectal cancer (CRC), commonly before age 50 years. The increased risk of synchronous and metachronous tumors raises the question of the optimal extent of resection at the time of initial diagnosis. When CRC is diagnosed, the surgeon is in the ideal position to order appropriate tumor testing for microsatellite instability (MSI) or immunohistochemical stains for loss of MMR gene associated protein, if this has not already been done. Part of the preoperative assessment should include careful consideration of the likelihood that HNPCC is present, as screening for extracolonic tumors may be warranted, recognizing the limited data regarding the utility of such investigations. A preoperative conclusion that HNPCC is definitely or likely present may lead to consideration of prophylactic hysterectomy/oophorectomy, because endometrial cancer is the second most common tumor in HNPCC, and ovarian cancer, though associated with less than a 10% lifetime risk in HNPCC carriers, carries a high mortality.

This article emphasizes the role of the 2 most commonly encountered of the genes responsible for HNPCC, namely *hMSH2* and *hMLH1*. It is not always possible to

Department of Gastrointestinal Medicine and Nutrition, University of Texas M. D. Anderson Cancer Center, 1515 Holcombe Boulevard, Box 436, Houston, TX 77030, USA
E-mail address: plynch@mdanderson.org

Surg Oncol Clin N Am 18 (2009) 611–624
doi:10.1016/j.soc.2009.08.002
1055-3207/09/$ – see front matter © 2009 Elsevier Inc. All rights reserved.

discuss these specific genes without commenting on the broader problem of HNPCC diagnosis and management.

Discovery of the first gene locus involved in HNPCC was a seminal event, as it confirmed that HNPCC was an actual disease entity.[1] Follow-up studies soon opened the door to recognition that HNPCC was due to mutations in one of several MMR genes, with defects in the function of these genes in turn responsible for the key molecular fingerprint in tumors, MSI.[2] That CRCs with MSI occur not only in HNPCC but in up to 15% of nonfamilial or sporadic CRCs demonstrates the wider importance of the so-called MSI pathway.[3,4] The improved prognoses of MSI tumors, accompanied by relative resistance to conventional chemotherapy drugs, have opened up a whole new area of interest for CRC biologists.[5] Meanwhile, a positive feedback loop exists in which advances in tumor biology and molecular genetics have clarified the importance of certain clinical-pathologic features. All of this has simplified some elements of the clinical approach to patients suspected of having HNPCC, while at the same time exasperating practitioners by enabling and thus ultimately forcing a more nuanced approach to patients with CRC.

This article reviews the history of HNPCC, its clinical features, gene discovery, development of clinical genetic workup, and clinical surveillance, with an emphasis on the 2 major HNPCC genes, hMSH2 and hMLH1. A companion article by Jenkins, elsewhere in this issue, addresses 2 other mismatch repair genes, hMSH6 and hPMS2.

HISTORY

HNPCC is also sometimes referred to as Lynch syndrome or Warthin-Lynch syndrome, after its early investigators. Family clusters of CRC uncomplicated by diffuse polyposis, and thus not a form of FAP, were described in the early 1900s.[6] For many decades it was not clear that HNPCC was a real entity at all, with some population genetics and epidemiology detractors arguing that familial clustering of CRC could be accounted for on the basis of chance aggregation alone. It was not until discovery of the first HNPCC locus in 1993 that HNPCC gained widespread acceptance as a bona fide disease.

In 1913, Warthin[6] reported one family with an excess of colorectal, gastric, and uterine cancer, describing it as a cancer family syndrome. The term "Cancer Family Syndrome" or "CFS" was actually in parlance for some years, being abandoned when it became evident that not only did the term convey little useful information, but that several other "Cancer Family Syndromes" existed that had nothing to do with CRC.[7]

In the 1960s Henry Lynch, assisted by Anne Krush, reported updated information about the original family "G" of Warthin and several additional families with similar features.[7–9] This series of articles, with additional reports by other investigators, eventually led to an agreed upon set of clinical features, the so-called Amsterdam Criteria (AC) for HNPCC.[10] These criteria included familial clustering of CRC (3 or more being required by the AC criteria, occurring over at least 2 generations) with at least one case showing early age at onset (age <50 years). Although Attenuated FAP (AFAP) was only starting to be clearly characterized at that time,[11,12] the framers of the AC wisely required that FAP and its variants be excluded. Over time, the importance of extracolonic tumors was recognized, especially endometrial cancer, and a revised set of Amsterdam Criteria, the AC-II, were adopted, in which one or more extracolonic tumors could be substituted for one or more cases of CRC in a given family pedigree.[13] The relatively stringent AC were adopted in part to provide specificity in the diagnosis of HNPCC in order that there would be confidence in recommending rigorous surveillance to close relatives of selected CRC patients. The AC were also used, again because of their stringency, as a basis for selection of kindreds on which to conduct linkage studies in search of an "HNPCC gene."

Initial efforts to find an HNPCC gene, shortly after the identification of the *APC* gene for FAP (1988–1990), were based on consideration of candidate genes such as *APC*, p53, and DCC. When the candidate gene approach bore no fruit, a genome-wide search was undertaken. In 1993, Peltomaki, Aaltonen, and colleagues, working in Helsinki, Finland, made 2 major discoveries contemporaneously. One was that there existed linkage between a locus on chromosome 2p and CRC in large Finnish HNPCC kindreds. The other was that tumors from most HNPCC patients showed evidence of a widespread "replication error phenotype" or "RER." It then became clear that these replication errors tended to involve microsatellite regions of genes, and that correction of such errors was under the control of a family of genes, already well characterized in yeast and other lower species. The term eventually accepted for the somatic mutations acquired in microsatellite regions of certain genes in HNPCC tumors was "microsatellite instability" or MSI. As with many other features of tumor biology, this was not a straightforward or consistent feature, as there is variability in the presence of MSI from tumor to tumor, along with variable susceptibility to mutation in microsatellites from gene to gene.

MUTATION TESTING

The sequences of the *hMSH2* and *hMLH1* genes are known. As in the case of *APC*, the genes are large and the number of deleterious mutations that may occur is large. Although there are some mutations that commonly recur as well as founder mutations that are frequent in a given geography or ethnic group, any given patient and family may have a truncating mutation that is unique and never described previously. Early on, it was thought that a relatively "simple" protein truncation assay or "PTT" would be useful for mutation detection. However, it soon became evident that many disease-causing mutations are not detected with such an assay. For this reason, end-to-end sequencing or sequence-sensitive assays are now employed in commercial laboratories in the United States and other countries.

As carefully selected cases, those with MSI or AC, were evaluated, it appeared that even the most rigorous end-to-end sequencing of *hMSH2* and *hMLH1* failed to detect mutations in roughly half of the cases tested. It turns out that some of the mutations that occur in *hMSH2* and *hMLH1* are large deletions that are not detected with existing mutation testing methods.[14] Southern blotting or, more recently, multiplex ligation-dependent probe amplification (MLPA), are used to detect such deletions, and these methods are now employed in commercial laboratories on failure of sequencing or denaturing high-performance liquid chromatography to detect HNPCC mutations. These measures have increased the mutation detection yield to nearly 70% in highly selected test populations.

Another approach to the problem of limited sensitivity of traditional testing has been the development of a so-called conversion assay, which separates maternal and paternal alleles for single strand analysis.[15,16] Although arguably increasing the mutation detection yield, to date this assay is difficult to perform and has not made its way into widespread clinical use.

One problematic category of mutation involves germline epigenetic silencing of *hMLH1* and less often *hMSH2*, based on methylation. Although this has been described in several families,[17–19] transmission over multiple generations is less likely to be maintained, due to the unstable nature of the mutation itself.[19]

VARIANTS OF UNCERTAIN SIGNIFICANCE

A major problem in dealing with "mutation" in these genes is the frequent occurrence of "variants of uncertain significance" (VUS), terms that commonly appear on reports from clinical genetic testing laboratories. Not all mutations in these genes cause truncation of the resultant protein so as to obviously compromise protein binding or function otherwise.[20] Yet sequence analysis will commonly show variants that are not clearly harmless polymorphisms. Considerable attention is being devoted to measures intended to properly classify such variants, including the development of functional assays.[21-23] As many as two-thirds of all variants found in one series were found to be a VUS.[23] Certain arbitrary criteria have been used to classify probability that a given VUS is in fact pathologic: Did the variant occur in multiple affected family members? Did it occur in and only in patients whose tumors showed MSI? Is the variant conserved across species? Does it affect a functional assay? Does the change in nucleotide sequence alter the amino acid sequence and does it affect protein structure in a manner likely to affect function?[24,25] To the extent that such information is provided as part of the variant description reported to a large database, it can strengthen the case for reclassifying the variant.

POPULATION VARIATION AND FOUNDER MUTATIONS

Early in the testing of suspected HNPCC subjects it became evident that some mutations were found repeatedly. Some evidently represented recurrent mutations in unrelated individuals. In other instances they were founder mutations, mutations that occurred many hundreds of years ago and were simply passed down for many generations. The earliest of these to be discovered, and among the most ancient, is likely the so-called Finnish mutation.[26,27] This mutation accounts for a large proportion of HNPCC cases in Finland. As such it provides an opportunity to initiate HNPCC mutation testing with simple "single site" testing which, if informative, is inexpensive and avoids the need for full-length sequencing and rearrangement studies of one or more MMR genes. Such founder mutations have been found in several other countries, mostly those whose populations have been fairly stable for long periods of time.[28-33] It therefore came as a surprise when a large number of recurring mutations in the heterogeneous population of the United States were traceable to a common ancestor.[34]

BIOLOGY OF hMSH2 AND hMLH1

The first 2 MMR genes to be identified, hMSH2 and hMLH1, encode proteins that are critical to the proper repair of DNA sequence mismatch, based on either single-base substitutions or insertion/deletion loops, reviewed recently by Seifert and Reichrath.[35] This DNA damage-repair system is highly conserved, indicating its importance and success in the evolutionary process. Study of mismatch repair in yeast species and in Escherichia coli provided the basis for the rapid understanding of the process in humans. Each of these proteins forms a heterodimer with its "minor" partners, hMSH2 with hMSH6 (and to a lesser extent with hMSH3), and hMLH1 with hPMS2 associated proteins. It seems that hMSH2 protein and its partners are involved in mismatch recognition, with hMLH1 combining in a ternary complex to facilitate strand excision.[36,37] There have been several useful reviews of the biology of MMR, including its specific role in HNPCC.[38,39] Although beyond the scope of this article, perturbation of MMR, whether occurring in HNPCC or sporadically, seems to have a bearing on prognosis and response of colorectal tumors to chemotherapeutic agents.[5,40-42]

ROLE OF MICROSATELLITE TESTING AND IMMUNOHISTOCHEMISTRY

The main practical advantage of identifying and sequencing the genes responsible for HNPCC was the ability to confirm that a given case of CRC was, in fact, HNPCC, and to establish a basis for performing predictive testing in at-risk relatives. It soon became evident that as many as half of all highly selected (ie, AC+) cases did not have a detectable mutation. It is now known that some AC+ cases lack MSI, and such families are, for now, termed "Familial Colon Cancer X" families[43] (see the article elsewhere in this issue by Lindor). An absence of MSI carries a very strong negative predictive value for MMR gene mutation detection. In contrast, excepting those cases that have somatically acquired MSI due to hMLH1 hypermethylation, evidence of high levels of MSI in a CRC predicts the presence of an MMR germline mutation in as many as 70% of cases. This situation is not ideal but does make a strong case for a stepwise approach to mutational testing (see articles in this issue by Aronson and Hempel).

Several important population studies have provided evidence of the potential importance of performing MSI testing before germline mutation testing. Before reviewing these, it is important to emphasize that no study to date has performed comprehensive mutational testing on *all* cases of CRC comprising a particular series, tending to avoid or at least limit testing in cases lacking MSI. Put another way, all cases undergoing mutational testing will have been enriched for mutation likelihood in one way or another.

The first important population study was that of Aaltonen and colleagues.[3] More than 500 consecutive cases in Finland were subjected to MSI testing with 7 markers. In cases showing MSI, mutation testing was performed for *hMSH2* and *hMLH1* mutations using 2-dimensional denaturing gradient gel electrophoresis or direct sequencing. Cases not showing MSI were tested only for the common Finnish founder mutation (exon 16 deletion in *hMLH1*). Overall, 12% of cases showed MSI, with 2% of the total having deleterious germline mutations, half of them being the Finnish founder mutation. Nine of the 10 mutation-positive cases had a colon or endometrial cancer-affected first-degree relative, and 4 of the 10 met AC for HNPCC. None of the MSI-stable cases had a mutation, but again only the common Finnish founder mutation was assayed. Of those cases with MSI but with no mutation detected, none had an immediate family history of CRC. One suspects that these were mostly, if not all, cases of hypermethylation. The investigators concluded that MSI testing has a powerful role in selecting cases for mutational testing, cautioning that most cases found to have MSI would have been identified anyway through clinical selection (positive family history, early onset, multiple primaries).

A more recent study from Spain[44] took a more direct look at several of the clinical predictors suggested by Aaltonen, which had by now been "codified" as the Bethesda guidelines,[45,46] and related these to both MSI and immunohistochemistry (IHC) for MMR-associated protein expression. Pinol and colleagues[44] collected nearly 2000 cases from 25 centers in Spain as part of the EPICOLON study. About 1200 were fully evaluable for tumor assay (including MSI, using only the *BAT26* marker, and IHC against MLH1 and MSH2 protein), germline mutation testing (sequencing and MLPA), and epidemiology assessment. Whereas only about 2% of cases met the AC, 23% met one or more of the Bethesda guidelines. MSI or protein expression loss by IHC was found in 91 of the 1222 evaluable cases (7.4%). Among these, 83 (6.8%) had MSI and 81 (6.6%) had loss of staining for MSH2 (21 cases) or MLH1 (60 cases) protein. Although nearly 90% concordance was shown between MSI and IHC, 10 cases had only MSI and 8 only an IHC abnormality, indicating a potential advantage of using both assays in a complementary fashion. Germline mutations were found in 11 cases (7 *hMSH2* and 4 *hMLH1*), or 0.9% of the total CRC population. As such, it is notable that for MSH2, 7 mutations were found among 21 cases with loss of MSH2 protein, whereas only 4 mutations were found in 60 cases showing loss of MLH1. This result offers further evidence that loss of MLH1, especially when occurring in an unselected population study, carries a much lower predictive power for mutation than does loss of MSH2, with most of this discrepancy due to somatic hypermethylation of the MLH1 promoter. As with the Aaltonen series, methylation assays were not conducted. Fulfillment of revised Bethesda guidelines alone carried a 3.5% positive predictive value (PPV) for mutation detection, whereas MSI and protein loss by IHC carried a 12% and 11% PPV, respectively. The absence of Bethesda guidelines, MSI, or IHC each carried at least a 99.9% negative predictive value. When Bethesda guidelines were combined with MSI or IHC, the PPV for mutation increased to 27% and 29%, respectively. The investigators concluded that adherence to Bethesda guidelines and use of MSI or IHC was a cost-effective strategy in working up patients with CRC. Limitations in the study were that comprehensive mutational testing was not done on cases lacking MSI or IHC abnormalities, and neither *hMSH6* or *hPMS2* were assessed.

The one North American population study was that of Hampel and colleagues,[47] conducted in Columbus, Ohio. The sample was intermediate in size between the Finnish and Spanish studies, but was in a sense the most "current" in that it did include methylation assay for cases showing MSI and it did evaluate for mutations in *hMSH6* and *hPMS2*. A slightly higher rate of high levels of MSI (MSI-H) was found, at 12.7%, and deleterious mutations were found in 2.2%. IHC was not done in all cases, but rather was limited to MSI cases and to those lacking MSI, but considered high probability based on clinical grounds. Of 135 MSI-H cases, 106 showed MLH1 promoter hypermethylation. This proportion, if applied in the Pinol series,[44] would have essentially accounted for the difference in mutation yield between the cases showing loss of MLH1 and MSH2; it also makes an argument favoring methylation testing in cases showing MLH1 loss. The investigators conclude that: MSI and IHC are valuable tools in selecting cases for mutation testing; MSI and IHC can be used more or less interchangeably; and technical problems in both MSI and IHC do exist and must be considered in deciding to routinely employ both assays.

Lindor and colleagues[48] had biospecimens from more than 1000 CRC cases, many but not all of which were retrieved from population-based collections. MSI analysis was performed with either 6 or 10 markers, and IHC against MLH1 and MSH2 proteins were done. More than 30% of cases showed MSI at 30% or more of the markers employed. Of these, 92% had a correspondingly informative IHC. Of cases showing protein loss, about 71% showed loss of MLH1 protein and 29% loss of MSH2. No cases that were microsatellite stable (MSS) or that had low levels of MSI (MSI-L) showed loss of protein staining. More recent population studies in the United States and Spain were able to evaluate subjects more comprehensively. Both the Pinol and Hampel studies[44,47] were able to take a more unbiased look at the relationship between MSI testing and IHC.

A few comments regarding technical limitations and issues in the performance of tissue-based evaluations are warranted. Several excellent recent reviews are available.[4]

Limitations of Microsatellite Instability Testing

Because MSI in a given gene sequence represents an acquired somatic mutation in tumor tissue, it constitutes a departure from normal DNA. To evaluate a microsatellite marker, one generally needs to compare the sequence variant with a source of normal

DNA. Although one could use blood as a source of genomic DNA, the anatomic pathologist finds normal mucosa easier to access. Surgical margins or otherwise uninvolved mucosa can be used. Endoscopic samples may be more likely to contain only tumor tissue. As such, a positive effort needs to be made to obtain normal mucosa. In the author's experience, simply sampling an area of uninvolved mucosa works well. There is evidence that there are several quasi-monomorphic mononucleotide microsatellite markers (BAT-26, BAT-25, NR-21, NR-22, NR-24), whose use may render unnecessary the acquisition of normal tissue as an internal normal reference. In this approach, maternal and paternal alleles will generally be represented as a single band, with the mutated allele from tumor comprising the only additional band.

Limitations of Immunohistochemistry

In evaluating tissue sections for expression of proteins associated with the respective MMR genes, several considerations must be kept in mind by the pathologist. The most important is the selection of the proper antibodies. Related to this is the importance of having proper positive and negative controls. In addition, it is important to be aware of the patterns of loss that occur. Because of the nature of the functional complexing of MSH2 and MSH6 proteins, a mutation in the hMSH2 gene, with resultant loss of MSH2 protein expression, will be associated with the additional loss of MSH6 protein. The converse, however, is not the case, so a mutation in hMSH6 will be associated only with loss of the MSH6 protein, with retained normal expression of MSH2 protein. When MLH1 is mutated, similarly both MLH1 and PMS2 expression will be lost. Yet an hPMS2 mutation and resultant loss of PMS2 expression immunohistochemically will not affect MLH1 protein expression.

Various technical considerations can account for lack of concordance between MSI testing and IHC. Some have to do with limitations in MSI assays, including for example the inability of dinucleotide markers to show instability in cases in which mononucleotide markers are informative.[49,50] In other instances the limitation may exist in the IHC technique.[51] Problems with fixation and staining can account for some of the variance. In other cases, variation in staining from one part of a tumor to another can be called "lack of staining" by one pathologist and "presence of staining" by another. Such cases may reflect actual heterogeneity of protein expression within the tumor, variation due to processing, fixation, and staining technique, or even variation in experience on the part of the interpreting pathologist. In addition, it is now known that pathogenic mutation in the *hMLH1* gene is not invariably associated with complete loss of protein expression.[52–55]

Limitations of Methylation Assays

Depending on the stringency in clinical criteria used to select cases for MSI testing, a case may be more likely to have MSI that reflects HNPCC (early onset, multiple primary or extracolonic HNPCC-associated tumors, family history) or that is in fact sporadic (older, R sided, poorly differentiated, or mucinous). As noted elsewhere, further evaluation of immunohistochemical staining patterns may (loss of hMSH2) or may not (loss of hMLH1) be specific for HNPCC. In cases that have both MSI and hMLH1 loss, there thus remains a real likelihood that germline testing will not be fruitful because the tumor is sporadic. The larger population studies[44,47] have amply demonstrated this point, with very large proportions of MSI/hMLH1 loss cases being shown to be sporadic. As alluded to elsewhere, it is now known that these changes are due to epigenetic silencing of hMLH1 by means of hypermethylation of its promoter. It suffices for the purposes of this discussion that the surgeon be aware that this phenomenon exists and that there are measures that can be employed to distinguish sporadic MSI from MSI due to HNPCC mutations. Complicating matters further is the observation of familial occurrences of hypermethylation of the *hMLH1* promoter. Thus, demonstration of hypermethylation may not invariably exclude the presence of an HNPCC mutation.[56] Assays to detect the presence of hypermethylation do exist and testing for presence of *BRAF* mutations can be employed.[56–59] Mutations in *BRAF* were initially seen as a feature distinguishing MSI from MSS tumors. It was later found that *BRAF* mutations are rarely, if ever, found in tumors from HNPCC patients.[60] Thus a fairly simple test for *BRAF* mutation in subjects with MSI or loss of hMLH1 expression can, when negative, provide strong evidence in support of the presence of HNPCC.[61–64] Efforts to find simpler means of performing *BRAF* testing have been under development.[65]

GENOTYPE-PHENOTYPE CORRELATIONS

A logical question for the surgeon to ask is whether, having found an *hMSH2* or *hMLH1* mutation, any clinically relevant differences in risk exist, depending on which gene is mutated or perhaps even on the location of the mutation in the particular gene. There is some evidence that differences in clinical expression exist between patients with mutations in *hMLH1* versus *hMSH2*. As with other types of studies in this area, the circumstances of subject selection and testing are important, and are summarized in enough detail to allow the reader to properly critique the work.

Goecke and colleagues[66] reported data from a German consortium and its experience with cases selected for HNPCC testing. Included were subjects with modified AC, personal history of 2 or more HNPCC-associated tumors, or early-onset CRC (age <45 years) or adenoma (age <40 years). Mutations were identified in slightly less than 50% of cases tested. It is worth noting that these were carefully selected, in most instances showed MSI or loss of MMR protein expression, and could be subjected to rearrangement studies in about half of the study centers. CRC occurred significantly more commonly in hMLH1 carriers (78%) than in hMSH2 carriers (65%), with lower rates for women than men with mutations in either gene. Significantly earlier overall (40 vs 43 years) and CRC-specific (41 vs 44 years) onset was seen in hMLH1 carriers compared with hMSH2 carriers. Significantly more CRCs were seen in hMLH1 families than in hMSH2. Although significantly more extracolonic HNPCC-associated tumors were seen in hMSH2 families, the only individual excess was nonmelanoma skin cancers (mainly of sebaceous differentiation), seen in hMSH2. No significant differences were otherwise seen with respect to individual extracolonic tumors, including endometrial.

Kastrinos and colleagues[67] evaluated nearly 2000 subjects, whose samples were submitted to a large United States commercial testing laboratory (Myriad Genetics) for HNPCC mutation testing. Sequencing alone was performed on approximately the first 900 cases while sequencing and genomic rearrangement studies were conducted on the most recent 1000 cases. Methylation testing that might have detected likely sporadic cases submitted on the basis of MSI or MLH1 protein loss was not performed. Indeed, because the testing laboratory does not perform MSI or IHC, it is not known what proportion of cases had previous tumor studies conducted. Keeping in mind the absence of rigorous criteria for submitting samples for testing, only about 15% of cases yielded pathologic mutations (12 in *hMLH1* and 173 in *hMSH2*), although 34% of cases meeting modified AC were found to have a mutation. Carriers of *hMSH2* mutations were more likely to have families meeting AC than were *hMLH1* carriers. Although the differences were not statistically significant, *hMLH1* carriers were more likely to have had CRC or to have had CRC only. These subjects were significantly younger than *hMSH2* carriers (42.2 years vs 44.8 years), a difference that was significant in men (38 vs 44 years) but not women. Subjects with *hMLH1* mutations had, on average, more CRCs in their families, and at an earlier age than *hMSH2* carriers. In the case of women, 9% had a history of endometrial cancer only. There was a moderately higher likelihood of having an *hMSH2* mutation detected, but no difference in age at diagnosis or strength of family history of endometrial cancer was found. Consistent with other reports, *hMSH2* carriers were significantly more likely to have various extracolonic HNPCC tumors, particularly sebaceous skin tumors, uroepithelial tumors, and ovarian cancers. Several other similar series have been published, with similar overall findings of greater CRC risk, earlier CRC onset, but fewer extracolonic tumors in *hMLH1* carriers relative to *hMSH2*.[68–74]

SUMMARY

The hMSH2 and hMLH1 genes are the most commonly mutated genes responsible for HNPCC. Key considerations to keep in mind in considering patients potentially affected with HNPCC include:

1. Recognize key clinical presenting features of patients with possible HNPCC, notably early age at onset, right colon involvement, characteristic pathology, and personal or family history of CRC or other HNPCC-associated tumors.
2. Have a low threshold for performing MSI or IHC evaluation on such patients, ideally at the time of diagnosis and before surgery An informative finding may alter the approach to surgical resection, even if germline mutational testing has not yet been performed or is uninformative; consider subtotal colectomy and total abdominal hysterectomy with bilateral salpingo-oopherectomy instead of simple segmental resection.
3. Be familiar with the sensitivities and specificities of MSI, IHC, and germline testing, and appreciate the problems of false positives (MSI that might be sporadic) and false negatives (uninformative germline testing). Reliance on genetic counselors and referral centers more familiar with the nuances of these issues may be helpful (see articles in this issue by Aronson and Hampel).
4. Understand that a positive germline test will usually carry greater significance in establishing a basis for predictive testing in at-risk relatives than it will in affecting management of the primary CRC patient.

Investigations in the near future will hopefully shed more light on specific genotype-phenotype correlations, improved assays for germline mutation detection (to reduce nondiagnostic tests), better functional assays to determine the relevance of sequence variants that are otherwise of uncertain significance, and attention to alterations in other genes that affect severity of expression in subjects with pathologic mutations in the genes of major interest. Unfortunately, most of the potential to be gained by such technical advances will have been wasted if practitioners are unable to motivate their patients to take advantage of them. More work will be required to overcome financial, psychological, and cultural barriers to the uptake of genetic testing and the screening/therapeutic measures enabled by such testing.

REFERENCES

1. Peltomaki P, Aaltonen LA, Sistonen P, et al. Genetic mapping of a locus predisposing to human colorectal cancer. Science 1993;260:810–2.

2. Peltomaki P, Lothe RA, Aaltonen LA, et al. Microsatellite instability is associated with tumors that characterize the hereditary non-polyposis colorectal carcinoma syndrome. Cancer Res 1993;53:5853–5.

3. Aaltonen LA, Salovaara R, Kristo P, et al. Incidence of hereditary nonpolyposis colorectal cancer and the feasibility of molecular screening for the disease. N Engl J Med 1998;338:1481–7.

4. Imai K, Yamamoto H. Carcinogenesis and microsatellite instability: the interrelationship between genetics and epigenetics. Carcinogenesis 2008;29: 673–80.

5. Ribic CM, Sargent DJ, Moore MJ, et al. Tumor microsatellite-instability status as a predictor of benefit from fluorouracil-based adjuvant chemotherapy for colon cancer. N Engl J Mod 2003;349;247–57.

6. Warthin A. Heredity with reference to carcinoma. Arch Intorn Med 1913;12: 546–55.

7. Lynch HT, Shaw MW, Magnuson CW, et al. Hereditary factors in cancer. Study of two large midwestern kindreds. Arch Intern Med 1966;117:206–12.

8. Lynch HT, Krush AJ. Heredity and adenocarcinoma of the colon. Gastroenterology 1967;53:517–27.

9. Lynch HT, Krush AJ, Larsen AL. Heredity and multiple primary malignant neoplasms: six cancer families. Am J Med Sci 1967;254:322–9.

10. Vasen HF, Mecklin JP, Khan PM, et al. The International Collaborative Group on Hereditary Non-Polyposis Colorectal Cancer (ICG-HNPCC). Dis Colon Rectum 1991;34:424–5.

11. Leppert M, Burt R, Hughes JP, et al. Genetic analysis of an inherited predisposition to colon cancer in a family with a variable number of adenomatous polyps. N Engl J Med 1990;322:904–8.

12. Spirio L, Olschwang S, Groden J, et al. Alleles of the APC gene: an attenuated form of familial polyposis. Cell 1993;75:951–7.

13. Vasen HF, Watson P, Mecklin JP, et al. New clinical criteria for hereditary nonpolyposis colorectal cancer (HNPCC, Lynch syndrome) proposed by the International Collaborative group on HNPCC. Gastroenterology 1999;116: 1453–6.

14. Nakagawa H, Hampel H, de la Chapelle A. Identification and characterization of genomic rearrangements of MSH2 and MLH1 in Lynch syndrome (HNPCC) by novel techniques. Hum Mutat 2003;22:258.

15. Nakagawa H, Yan H, Lockman J, et al. Allele separation facilitates interpretation of potential splicing alterations and genomic rearrangements. Cancer Res 2002; 62:4579–82.

16. Casey G, Lindor NM, Papadopoulos N, et al. Conversion analysis for mutation detection in MLH1 and MSH2 in patients with colorectal cancer. JAMA 2005; 293:799–809.

17. Suter CM, Martin DI, Ward RL. Germline epimutation of MLH1 in individuals with multiple cancers. Nat Genet 2004;36:497–501.

18. Chan TL, Yuen ST, Kong CK, et al. Heritable germline epimutation of MSH2 in a family with hereditary nonpolyposis colorectal cancer. Nat Genet 2006;38: 1178–83.

19. Hitchins MP, Wong JJ, Suthers G, et al. Inheritance of a cancer-associated MLH1 germ-line epimutation. N Engl J Med 2007;356:697–705.

20. Ollila S, Sarantaus L, Kariola R, et al. Pathogenicity of MSH2 missense mutations is typically associated with impaired repair capability of the mutated protein. Gastroenterology 2006;131:1408–17.

21. Belvederesi L, Bianchi F, Galizia E, et al. MSH2 missense mutations and HNPCC syndrome: pathogenicity assessment in a human expression system. Hum Mutat 2008;29:E296–309.
22. Belvederesi L, Bianchi F, Loretelli C, et al. Assessing the pathogenicity of MLH1 missense mutations in patients with suspected hereditary nonpolyposis colorectal cancer: correlation with clinical, genetic and functional features. Eur J Hum Genet 2006;14:853–9.
23. Barnetson RA, Cartwright N, van Vliet A, et al. Classification of ambiguous mutations in DNA mismatch repair genes identified in a population-based study of colorectal cancer. Hum Mutat 2008;29:367–74.
24. Ng PC, Henikoff S. Predicting deleterious amino acid substitutions. Genome Res 2001;11:863–74.
25. Ng PC, Henikoff S. Predicting the effects of amino acid substitutions on protein function. Annu Rev Genomics Hum Genet 2006;7:61–80.
26. Nystrom-Lahti M, Kristo P, Nicolaides NC, et al. Founding mutations and Alu-mediated recombination in hereditary colon cancer. Nat Med 1995;1:1203–6.
27. de la Chapelle A, Wright FA. Linkage disequilibrium mapping in isolated populations: the example of Finland revisited. Proc Natl Acad Sci U S A 1998;95: 12416–23.
28. Nilbert M, Wikman FP, Hansen TV, et al. Major contribution from recurrent alterations and MSH6 mutations in the Danish Lynch syndrome population. Fam Cancer 2009;8:75–83.
29. Yap HL, Chieng WS, Lim JR, et al. Recurring MLH1 deleterious mutations in unrelated Chinese Lynch syndrome families in Singapore. Fam Cancer 2008; 8:85–94.
30. de Leon MP, Benatti P, Di Gregorio C, et al. Genotype-phenotype correlations in individuals with a founder mutation in the MLH1 gene and hereditary non-polyposis colorectal cancer. Scand J Gastroenterol 2007;42:746–53.
31. Sun S, Greenwood CM, Thiffault I, et al. The HNPCC associated MSH2*1906G->C founder mutation probably originated between 1440 CE and 1715 CE in the Ashkenazi Jewish population. J Med Genet 2005;42:766–8.
32. Chan TL, Chan YW, Ho JW, et al. MSH2 c.1452-1455delAATG is a founder mutation and an important cause of hereditary nonpolyposis colorectal cancer in the southern Chinese population. Am J Hum Genet 2004;74:1035–42.
33. Buerstedde JM, Alday P, Torhorst J, et al. Detection of new mutations in six out of 10 Swiss HNPCC families by genomic sequencing of the hMSH2 and hMLH1 genes. J Med Genet 1995;32:909–12.
34. Lynch HT, Coronel SM, Okimoto R, et al. A founder mutation of the MSH2 gene and hereditary nonpolyposis colorectal cancer in the United States. JAMA 2004;291:718–24.
35. Seifert M, Reichrath J. The role of the human DNA mismatch repair gene hMSH2 in DNA repair, cell cycle control and apoptosis: implications for pathogenesis, progression and therapy of cancer. J Mol Histol 2006;37:301–7.
36. Galio L, Bouquet C, Brooks P. ATP hydrolysis-dependent formation of a dynamic ternary nucleoprotein complex with MutS and MutL. Nucleic Acids Res 1999;27: 2325–31.
37. Hall MC, Matson SW. The *Escherichia coli* MutL protein physically interacts with MutH and stimulates the MutH-associated endonuclease activity. J Biol Chem 1999;274:1306–12.
38. Peltomaki P. Role of DNA mismatch repair defects in the pathogenesis of human cancer. J Clin Oncol 2003;21:1174–9.

39. Modrich P. Mechanisms in eukaryotic mismatch repair. J Biol Chem 2006;281: 30305–9.

40. Vilar E, Scaltriti M, Balmana J, et al. Microsatellite instability due to hMLH1 deficiency is associated with increased cytotoxicity to irinotecan in human colorectal cancer cell lines. Br J Cancer 2008;99:1607–12.

41. Bertagnolli MM, Niedzwiecki D, Compton CC, et al. Microsatellite instability predicts improves response to adjuvant therapy with irinotecan, fluorouracil, and leucovorin in stage III colon cancer: Cancer and Leukemia Group B Protocol 89803. J Clin Oncol 2009;27:1814–21.

42. Kim GP, Colangelo LH, Wieand HS, et al. Prognostic and predictive roles of high-degree microsatellite instability in colon cancer: a National Cancer Institute-National Surgical Adjuvant Breast and Bowel Project Collaborative Study. J Clin Oncol 2007;25:767–72.

43. Lindor NM, Rabe K, Petersen GM, et al. Lower cancer incidence in Amsterdam-I criteria families without mismatch repair deficiency: familial colorectal cancer type X. JAMA 2005;293:1979–85.

44. Pinol V, Castells A, Andreu M, et al. Accuracy of revised Bethesda guidelines, microsatellite instability, and immunohistochemistry for the identification of patients with hereditary nonpolyposis colorectal cancer. JAMA 2005;293: 1986–94.

45. Rodriguez-Bigas MA, Boland CR, Hamilton SR, et al. A National Cancer Institute Workshop on Hereditary Nonpolyposis Colorectal Cancer Syndrome: meeting highlights and Bethesda guidelines. J Natl Cancer Inst 1997;89:1758–62.

46. Umar A, Boland CR, Terdiman JP, et al. Revised Bethesda Guidelines for hereditary nonpolyposis colorectal cancer (Lynch syndrome) and microsatellite instability. J Natl Cancer Inst 2004;96:261–8.

47. Hampel H, Frankel WL, Martin E, et al. Screening for the Lynch syndrome (hereditary nonpolyposis colorectal cancer). N Engl J Med 2005;352:1851–60.

48. Lindor NM, Burgart LJ, Leontovich O, et al. Immunohistochemistry versus microsatellite instability testing in phenotyping colorectal tumors. J Clin Oncol 2002;20: 1043–8.

49. Suraweera N, Duval A, Reperant M, et al. Evaluation of tumor microsatellite instability using 5 quasimonomorphic mononucleotide repeats and pentaplex PCR. Gastroenterology 2002;123:1804–11.

50. Buhard O, Suraweera N, Lectard A, et al. Quasimonomorphic mononucleotide repeats for high-level microsatellite instability analysis. Dis Markers 2004;20: 251–7.

51. Chapusot C, Martin L, Puig PL, et al. What is the best way to assess microsatellite instability status in colorectal cancer? Study on a population base of 462 colorectal cancers. Am J Surg Pathol 2004;28:1553–9.

52. Curia MC, Palmirotta R, Aceto G, et al. Unbalanced germ-line expression of hMLH1 and hMSH2 alleles in hereditary nonpolyposis colorectal cancer. Cancer Res 1999;59:3570–5.

53. Salahshor S, Koelble K, Rubio C, et al. Microsatellite Instability and hMLH1 and hMSH2 expression analysis in familial and sporadic colorectal cancer. Lab Invest 2001;81:535–41.

54. Thibodeau SN, French AJ, Cunningham JM, et al. Microsatellite instability in colorectal cancer: different mutator phenotypes and the principal involvement of hMLH1. Cancer Res 1998;58:1713–8.

55. Wahlberg SS, Schmeits J, Thomas G, et al. Evaluation of microsatellite instability and immunohistochemistry for the prediction of germ-line MSH2 and MLH1

mutations in hereditary nonpolyposis colon cancer families. Cancer Res 2002;62: 3485–92.

56. Cunningham JM, Christensen ER, Tester DJ, et al. Hypermethylation of the hMLH1 promoter in colon cancer with microsatellite instability. Cancer Res 1998;58:3455–60.

57. Kane MF, Loda M, Gaida GM, et al. Methylation of the hMLH1 promoter correlates with lack of expression of hMLH1 in sporadic colon tumors and mismatch repair-defective human tumor cell lines. Cancer Res 1997;57:808–11.

58. Deng G, Chen A, Hong J, et al. Methylation of CpG in a small region of the hMLH1 promoter invariably correlates with the absence of gene expression. Cancer Res 1999;59:2029–33.

59. Rajagopalan H, Bardelli A, Lengauer C, et al. Tumorigenesis: RAF/RAS oncogenes and mismatch-repair status. Nature 2002;418:934.

60. Deng G, Bell I, Crawley S, et al. BRAF mutation is frequently present in sporadic colorectal cancer with methylated hMLH1, but not in hereditary nonpolyposis colorectal cancer. Clin Cancer Res 2004;10:191–5.

61. Ogino S, Nosho K, Kirkner GJ, et al. CpG island methylator phenotype, microsatellite instability, BRAF mutation and clinical outcome in colon cancer. Gut 2009; 58:90–6.

62. Soreide K. Molecular testing for microsatellite instability and DNA mismatch repair defects in hereditary and sporadic colorectal cancers—ready for prime time? Tumour Biol 2007;28:290–300.

63. Boland CR. Clinical uses of microsatellite instability testing in colorectal cancer: an ongoing challenge. J Clin Oncol 2007;25:754–6.

64. Lynch HT, Boland CR, Rodriguez-Bigas MA, et al. Who should be sent for genetic testing in hereditary colorectal cancer syndromes? J Clin Oncol 2007;25: 3534–42.

65. Benlloch S, Paya A, Alenda C, et al. Detection of BRAF V600E mutation in colorectal cancer: comparison of automatic sequencing and real-time chemistry methodology. J Mol Diagn 2006;8:540–3.

66. Goecke T, Schulmann K, Engel C, et al. Genotype-phenotype comparison of German MLH1 and MSH2 mutation carriers clinically affected with Lynch syndrome: a report by the German HNPCC Consortium. J Clin Oncol 2006;24: 4285–92.

67. Kastrinos F, Stoffel EM, Balmana J, et al. Phenotype comparison of MLH1 and MSH2 mutation carriers in a cohort of 1,914 individuals undergoing clinical genetic testing in the United States. Cancer Epidemiol Biomarkers Prev 2008; 17:2044–51.

68. Vasen HF, Wijnen JT, Menko FH, et al. Cancer risk in families with hereditary nonpolyposis colorectal cancer diagnosed by mutation analysis. Gastroenterology 1996;110:1020–7.

69. Parc Y, Boisson C, Thomas G, et al. Cancer risk in 348 French MSH2 or MLH1 gene carriers. J Med Genet 2003;40:208–13.

70. Farrington SM, Lin-Goerke J, Ling J, et al. Systematic analysis of hMSH2 and hMLH1 in young colon cancer patients and controls. Am J Hum Genet 1998; 63:749–59.

71. Dunlop MG, Farrington SM, Carothers AD, et al. Cancer risk associated with germline DNA mismatch repair gene mutations. Hum Mol Genet 1997;6:105–10.

72. Bisgaard ML, Jager AC, Myrhoj T, et al. Hereditary non-polyposis colorectal cancer (HNPCC): phenotype-genotype correlation between patients with and without identified mutation. Hum Mutat 2002;20:20–7.

73. Vasen HF, Stormorken A, Menko FH, et al. MSH2 mutation carriers are at higher risk of cancer than MLH1 mutation carriers: a study of hereditary nonpolyposis colorectal cancer families. J Clin Oncol 2001;19:4074–80.

74. Peltomaki P, Gao X, Mecklin JP. Genotype and phenotype in hereditary nonpolyposis colon cancer: a study of families with different vs shared predisposing mutations. Fam Cancer 2001;1:9–15.

Role of MSH6 and PMS2 in the DNA Mismatch Repair Process and Carcinogenesis

Mark A. Jenkins, PhD

KEYWORDS

• MSH6 • PMS2 • Mismatch repair • Penetrance

The fidelity of DNA synthesis during cell replication is maintained by the mismatch repair system, which detects and repairs DNA mismatches—point mutations caused by base substitutions, insertions, or deletions.[1] Loss of mismatch repair function can result in the accrual of mismatches with subsequent replication leading to the mutator phenotype. Cancers consequent to this mutator phenotype are characterized by microsatellite instability (MSI) due to the inability of the mismatch repair system to repair commonly occurring mismatches in repeat sequences.

The mismatch repair system in humans and other eukaryotes is initiated by a heterodimer most commonly comprising MSH2 and MSH6 (MutSα), two mismatch repair proteins made by the mismatch repair genes *MSH2* and *MSH6* respectively. Once the MutSα heterodimer is bound to the mismatch, a second heterodimer (MutL), most commonly comprising MLH1 and PMS2, made by the genes *MLH1* and *PMS2*, interacts with MutSα to excise and repair the mismatch.[2]

Some DNA mismatches may be able to be repaired even in the absence of MSH6 or PMS2. Initiation of the mismatch repair process can be initiated with MutSβ, the heterodimer of MSH2 and MSH3, which can share the role of mismatch recognition with MutSα, especially of single-base insertions.[1] Similarly, a homolog of the MutL, MutLγ (MLH1–MLH3) is thought to repair insertions or deletions.[3] Therefore, some DNA mismatches may be repaired in the absence of MSH6 and PMS2.

Loss of mismatch repair function in a cell can occur via a variety of mechanisms, including germline mutation of a mismatch repair followed by somatic loss of the second allele or by somatic loss of both alleles. Somatic loss appears to be a function of age.

Centre for MEGA Epidemiology, School of Population Health, Level 1, 723 Swanston St, The University of Melbourne, Victoria 3010, Australia
E-mail address: m.jenkins@unimelb.edu.au

Surg Oncol Clin N Am 18 (2009) 625–636
doi:10.1016/j.soc.2009.07.007
1055-3207/09/$ – see front matter © 2009 Elsevier Inc. All rights reserved.

surgonc.theclinics.com

DISCOVERY OF INHERITED MUTATIONS IN *MSH6* AND *PMS2*

The first reports of inherited mutations in *MSH6* and *PMS2* were studies of DNA samples from colorectal cancer patients who had a strong family history of colorectal and other cancers, and in whom mutations in *MLH1* and *MSH2* could not be found.

The first reported inherited mutation in *MSH6* was identified in a Japanese woman diagnosed with colorectal cancer and endometrial cancer in her 50s. She had two sisters diagnosed with endometrial cancer, one sister with ovarian cancer, and a brother with pancreatic cancer, all diagnosed before age diagnosed 70.[4]

The first report of an inherited mutation in *PMS2* was identified in a cancer patient (site unreported) who had a family history of colorectal cancer meeting the Amsterdam criteria for HNPCC.[5]

NUMBER OF MUTATIONS IN *MSH6* AND *PMS2*

It is difficult to describe the spectrum of mutations in *MSH6* and *PMS2* because: (1) there are no "hotspots" as the variants are spread across the coding and regulatory regions of the genes; (2) it is often difficult to determine the pathogenicity of any variant; (3) many variants are not reported or published; and (4) use of nomenclature of genetic variants has been inconsistent.

There are several databases of genetic variants of mismatch repair genes. These include the Leiden Open Variation Database managed from Leiden University Medical Center (www.lovd.nl); the Mismatch Repair Genes Variant Database,[6] which is a database of "only those variants which have been published in peer-reviewed journals" using a standard nomenclature; and the MMR Gene Unclassified Variants database (www.mmrmissense.net/), which contains information from functional assays and other types of data to support the interpretation of the unclassified variants of the MMR gene. As of March 2009, the combined databases contained 377 distinct *MSH6* variants and 176 distinct variants in *PMS2* (as compared to 1004 for *MLH1* and 888 for *MSH2*). According to the Mismatch Repair Genes Variant Database,[6] of the *MSH6* variants, 37% were insertions/deletions, 27% were missense, 21% were silent, 11% were nonsense, 2% were large genomic deletions/duplications, and 2% were splicing variants. In contrast, for *PMS2*, the most commonly described variants were missense (49%), followed by large genomic deletions/duplications (19%), silent (15%), insertions/deletions (9%), and nonsense (7%).

The apparent lower proportion of mismatch repair gene mutations due to *PMS2* compared to the other mismatched repair genes may not be due to a lower mutation frequency. Testing for germline mutations in *PMS2* is not as straightforward as for *MSH6* or the other mismatch repair genes. There are at least 13 highly homologous *PMS2* pseudogenes, the majority of which have some homology with at least some of the 10 exons at the 3' end of the gene.[7–10] Long-range polymerase chain reaction, in which primers are selected from regions with no pseudogene homology, has been shown to avoid the amplification of pseudogene sequences.[11–13] Due to these issues, testing for *PMS2* has been limited to a few laboratories, possibly limiting the rate of testing and therefore identification of new mutations.

Although these databases describe the variety of variants identified in *MSH6* and *PMS2*, they do not provide information on the frequency of variants in the population. In the only published study to date reporting the estimated prevalence of mismatch repair gene mutations in the population, it is estimated that 1 in 3139 (95% CI, 1 in 1247 to 1 in 7626) 15- to 74-year-olds carry a mutation in *MLH1* or *MSH2*.[14] There have been no published estimates of the comparative figures for *MSH6* or *PMS2*.

MSH6 AND PMS2 AND CANCER

Mutations in mismatch repair genes have been shown to consistently result in a substantially increased risk of cancer in carriers. The degree to which cancer risk is increased for carriers of MSH6 and PMS2 is discussed in detail in the penetrance section below. The cancer risks are most substantially increased for cancer of the colon and rectum (colorectal) and cancer of the endometrium. Cancers of the small bowel, stomach, pancreas, ovary, renal pelvis, ureter, bladder, brain, appendix, liver, bile duct, gall bladder, and skin have also been reported to be at increased incidence in mismatch repair gene mutation carriers.[13] Cancers caused by mismatch repair gene mutation have been referred to as Lynch cancers, after Dr. Henry Lynch, who, before the identification of the mismatch repair genes, described the apparently dominantly inherited spectrum of cancers. Somewhat confusingly, this spectrum of cancers caused by MMR gene mutations has also been described as hereditary nonpolyposis colorectal cancer (HNPCC) despite many of the cancers being extracolonic. The term Lynch syndrome is becoming more acceptable now as a description of an individual with a cancer caused by a mismatch repair gene mutation, and the cancers that are at increased risk are termed Lynch syndrome cancers.[5]

Several population-based studies have reported the prevalence of MSH6 and PMS2 mutations in persons diagnosed with colorectal cancer and endometrial cancer (see **Table 1**). These studies suggest that, in individuals with cancer, mutations in MSH6 and PMS2 are less common than mutations in MLH1 and MSH2. In a population-based study of newly diagnosed colorectal cancer patients recruited, regardless of age or the presence or absence of a family history, from six participating hospitals in Ohio, investigators reported that 44 of 1566 colorectal cancer cases had a germline mutations in a DNA mismatch repair gene (2.8%; 95% CI, 2.1%–3.8%). Of these, 73% (n = 32) were either MLH1 or MSH2 compared with 14% (n = 6) for MSH6 and 14% (n = 6) for PMS2.[15,16] These data suggest that 0.4% of colorectal cancer cases arise because of germline mutations in MSH6, and the same proportion of colorectal cancers are due to PMS2 mutations.

The same group reported that of 543 endometrial cancers, 10 (1.8%) had germline mutations in an mismatch repair gene.[17] In endometrial cancers, in contrast to colorectal cancer, the minority of the mismatch repair gene mutations were MLH1 or

---

Table 1
Proportion (95% confidence intervals) of population-based colorectal and endometrial cancer cases identified as carriers of a deleterious germline mutation in MSH6 or PMS2

Age of Diagnosis	Proportion of Cases who are Carriers of MSH6 Mutations	Proportion of Cases who are Carriers of PMS2 Mutations
Colorectal cancer		
All ages	1 in 261 (1 in 121 to 1 in 711)[16,17]	1 in 261 (1 in 121 to 1 in 711)[16,17]
under 60 y	1 in 672 (1 in 186 to 1 in 5546)[2]	1 in 672 (1 in 186 to 1 in 5546)[2]
under 55 y	1 in 124 (1 in 61 to 1 in 309)[20]	No testing conducted
under 50 y	No carrier identified[16,18]	1 in 131 (1 in 37 to 1 in 1084)[16,18]
under 45 yrs	1 In 26 (1 in 11 to 1 in 95)[21]	No testing conducted
50+ y	1 in 217 (1 in 100 to 1 in 591)[16,18]	1 in 326 (1 in 128 to 1 in 1195)[16,18]
Endometrial cancer		
All ages	1 in 91 (1 in 42 to 1 in 246)[18]	No testing conducted
All ages	1 in 63 (1 in 31 to 1 in 156)[19]	No testing conducted

MSH2 (n = 4) with the majority (n = 6) having an *MSH6* mutation; there were no *PMS2* mutations detected. These data suggest that 1% of endometrial cancers arise from germline mutations in *MSH6*. Therefore, in comparison to colorectal cancer, endometrial cancers are approximately 2.5 times more likely to be due to *MSH6* mutations. A hospital series of 441 patients with endometrial cancers unselected for family history identified 7 (1.6%) who were *MSH6* mutation carriers.[18]

There is some evidence that the prevalence of *MSH6* mutations for colorectal cancer cases is higher for those diagnosed at an early age compared with those diagnosed at a later age. For example, a West Australian population-based study of colorectal cancers diagnosed under age 60 reported 0.15% were carriers of *MSH6* mutations.[2] A study of population-based colorectal cancers diagnosed before age 55 in Scotland reported that *MSH6* mutations accounted for 0.8% of colorectal cancer diagnosed before age 55,[19] and a study of population-based colorectal cancers diagnosed before age 45 in Melbourne, Australia, found that MSH6 mutations accounted for 3.8% of colorectal cancer diagnosed before age 45.[20] However, this inverse relationship with age of diagnosis has not been observed by all studies. In contrast, the Ohio study of a series of colorectal cancers (described above) found that all 6 cases with a *MSH6* mutation were diagnosed over the age of 50 (0.5%).

The equivalent age-specific data for *PMS2* mutations comes from the Ohio study, which identified 6 *PMS2* carriers using long-range polymerase chain reaction detection methods. Investigators observed that 0.8% of colorectal cancer cases diagnosed under 50 years were compared with 0.3% of colorectal cancer cases diagnosed aged 50 years or over.[15,17] A West Australian study of population-based colorectal cancers diagnosed under age 60 reported 0.15% were carriers of *PMS2* mutations.[2]

IDENTIFICATION OF CARRIERS OF *MSH6* AND *PMS2* MUTATIONS

Testing for mutations in mismatch repair genes, including *MSH6* and *PMS2*, is a time-consuming and human resource–intensive exercise because of the number of genes involved, the lack of any "hot spots" or common mutation-prohibiting predictive testing, the size of the genes, the pre- and posttest genetic counseling required, and the existence of pseudogenes for *PMS2* (see above). These issues make it impractical to test populations of unaffected individuals and may require, because of costs, testing of only cancer cases most likely to be carriers of mismatch repair mutations. Several criteria have been developed to identify sets of individuals most likely to have inherited a mismatch mutation and therefore most likely to benefit from mutation testing.

Family history of Lynch syndrome cancers have commonly been used to identify individuals with a sufficiently high probability of carrying an MMR gene mutation to warrant genetic testing. The commonly used criteria of family history of cancer to identify individuals to genetically test for MMR gene mutations was the modified Amsterdam criteria, later refined as the Amsterdam II criteria[21]: at least three relatives with cancer of the colorectum, endometrium, small bowel, ureter, or renal pelvis; with one of the relatives a first-degree relative of the other two; with involvement of at least two generations; with at least one case diagnosed before the age of 50; and without familial adenomatous polyposis.

An alternative method of identification of individuals at increased probability of carrying a MMR gene mutation—a method independent of family history of cancer—is a genetic test or pathology examination of the tumor for evidence of loss of mismatch repair. The two most widely used tests are: (1) a genetic test of MSI, a hallmark of loss of mismatch repair function; and (2) immounohistochemical (IHC) test of the tumor for presence of mismatch repair proteins. Individuals with a cancer that exhibits loss of mismatch repair function according to either test are not necessarily carriers of mismatch repair gene mutations (as loss may occur somatically only), but are at increased probability of having a mutation in the germline, particularly if diagnosed at an early age.[2,22]

MSH6

In the Ohio series of colorectal cancers described above, where subjects were unselected for family history of cancer, none of the six MSH6 mutation carriers had a family history meeting the Amsterdam II criteria but all six had colorectal cancer tumors that exhibited loss of MMR proteins by IHC and were MSI.[15,23] Therefore while MSI and IHC had 100% sensitivity for MSH6 mutations, Amsterdam criteria had 0% sensitivity. A further advantage of IHC over family history of cancer is that the genes to be tested for mutations can be inferred by which proteins are not being expressed. MSI testing can also imply which mismatch repair genes should be tested. A population-based study of early-onset colorectal cancer cases diagnosed before 45 years, tested all tumors for 15 microsatellite markers followed by germline testing for mismatch repair gene mutations. A panel of 10 markers, including 7 mononucleotide markers, could distinguish all three MSH6 mutation carriers, which all had colorectal cancer tumors that were MSI-low (instability in 2–5 of the 10 markers tested) from the 12 mLH1 and MSH2 carriers, which all had colorectal cancer tumors that were MSI-high (instability in 6–10 markers).[24]

PMS2

Individuals with colorectal cancer tumors with IHC showing loss of MLH1 and PMS2 are usually tested for mutations in MLH1 since previous studies suggest that an MLH1 mutation is more likely than a PMS2 mutation. However, isolated loss of PMS2 protein expression (defined as loss of PMS2 and retention of MLH1, MSH2, and MSH6), which occurs in 4.3% of colorectal tumors exhibiting a high degree of MSI (95% CI, 2.7%–6.4%),[25] is a strong predictor of a germline mutation in PMS2. A study of 99 tumors with isolated loss of PMS2 by IHC (91 colorectal, 5 endometrial, 1 transitional cell of the renal pelvis, 1 small intestinal, and 1 gastric) found that 61 of the cases (62%) were found to have deleterious germline mutations in the PMS2 and a further 10 had missense variants of unknown pathogenicity[26] (ie, a positive predictive value of 62%). In contrast, for 43 patients whose tumors also exhibited loss of MLH1, no PMS2 mutations were found, suggesting that, in practice, searching for PMS2 mutations should be limited to cases where PMS2 alone is not expressed in a tumor.

Once MMR mutation carriers are identified, predictive testing of relatives can be conducted for the same mutation identified in the proband.

RISK OF CANCER IN MSH6 AND PMS2 MUTATION CARRIERS (PENETRANCE)

Although carriers of MSH6 or PMS2 mutations are at substantially increased risk of cancer—as is the case for the MLH1 and MSH2 mutation carriers—penetrance is much lower than 100% (compare with familial adenomatous polyposis). Why some mutation carriers develop cancer, even at an early age, while other carriers remain cancer-free to old age is not known. Possible modifiers of genetic risk include the type of mutation, environmental exposures, and other genetic factors, although theoretically a distribution of risk exists because of the stochastic probability of the somatic loss of the functioning allele and the subsequent accrual of mutations due to unrepaired mismatches in subsequent generations of cells. In other words, given enough time, all carriers of mismatch repair carriers would eventually develop cancer and, on average, at a greater rate than noncarriers. This age-dependent risk function may depend on a number of factors, so there is not one penetrance. Even for carriers restricted to one gene (e.g. just *MSH6* carriers or just *PMS2* carriers), factors that may influence risk in mutation carriers include the type of mutation (e.g. protein-truncating, frameshift, missense, deletion, insertion); the site of the mutation (intronic, exonic, relationship to 3' and 5' ends); demographic, environmental, and lifestyle characteristics of the carrier (e.g. age, sex, anthropometry, dietary characteristics, hormone use, alcohol and smoking); and genotype of the carrier (e.g. variants in other modifier genes). Therefore, any particular study can at best only estimate an average risk for a set of mutations occurring in a given population setting, and it is not logical to refer to the penetrance of mismatch repair genes.

Because of the rarity of mutations in *MSH6* and *PMS2*, family studies have the most appropriate design to investigate risk of disease. The relatives of a mutation carrier that first brings their family to the attention of the investigator, the (proband) undergo predictive testing for the same mutation, thereby accruing carriers for a retrospective analysis of risk. Mutation-carrying families for penetrance studies have been ascertained by two general approaches: (1) via individuals who have sought genetic testing because of a family history of cancer (clinic-based ascertainment); or (2) via a cancer case identified from a population-based source (commonly a cancer registry) or a cancer series unselected because of family history of cancer (population-based ascertainment). Both are legitimate sources of individuals for penetrance analysis. However, estimates of penetrance must be conditioned on the method of ascertainment.

A potential consequence of not correctly conditioning on ascertainment, when estimating penetrance using families ascertained from family cancer clinics, is that estimates of risk are likely to be inflated. First, if testing for family-specific genetic mutations were to be systematically more likely in affected persons (i.e. cases) than in unaffected persons (controls), penetrance estimates would be biased upwards.[27] Second, because these families came into the study specifically because they had an overpreponderance of colorectal and perhaps related cancers, naïve analysis, as if the relatives are a random sample, will obviously result in a spuriously high estimate. Appropriate adjustment for sampling must be made, but this is not always straightforward. Estimates of mismatch repair gene mutation penetrance of families that have not correctly conditioned on ascertainment selected from family cancer clinics have been shown to be inflated approximately twofold.[28]

MSH6

Few studies have attempted to estimate penetrance for *MSH6* mutations, so knowledge of the consequences of such mutations remains uncertain (see **Table 2**).

Three studies have analyzed cancer risk in *MSH6* mutation carriers ascertained from families referred to clinics because of family history of colorectal or other cancers. All used the Kaplan–Meier survival analysis method to estimate the cumulative risk of cancer. However, none conditioned on the ascertainment criteria of family history of cancer, so estimates are likely to be biased upwards (ie, inflated).[28] A study of 146 *MSH6* mutation carriers identified from 20 families referred because of family history of colorectal cancer[29] estimated colorectal cancer risk to age 70 as 69% for men and 30% for women. The estimate of 71% cumulative risk to age 70 of endometrial cancer is less likely to be biased because the carriers in this study do not appear to

Table 2
Cumulative risk of cancer in carriers of germline mutations in *MSH6* and *PMS2* by study, country, ascertainment, and number of carriers

Gene	Country	Ascertainment	Carriers (Families)	Cumulative Risk to Age 70
MSH6	The Netherlands[29]	Clinic-based (FH CRC and Am I)	146 (20)	CRC men: 69% (42%–83%)[a] CRC women: 30% (12%–44%)[a] EC: 71% (50%–83%)
MSH6	Germany[31]	Clinic-based (Am II)	70 (27)	CRC men and women: 80%[a]
MSH6	Sweden[33]	Population-based (double primary CRC, EC)	23 (7)	CRC men and women: 33%[a] EC: 65%[a] LS males: 25%[a] LS females: 85%[a] EC: 70% (49%–91%)[a]
MSH6	United States[34]	Population-based (EC all ages)	59 (7)	Any cancers: 37% CRC men and women: 25% (0%–70%)[37] EC: 20% (5%–42%)[37]
MSH6	Australia[35]	Population-based (CRC under age 45)	20 (4)	CRC men and women: 45% (25%–70%)[37] EC: 40% (15%–65%)[37]
MSH6	United States, Canada, Australia, Netherlands, Scotland[37]	Population-based (CRC at various ages) and from clinic-based (Am II)	1043 (113)	CRC males: 22% (14%–32%) CRC females: 10% (5%–17%) EC: 26% (18%–36%) LS males: 24% (16%–37%) LS females: 40% (32%–52%)
PMS2	United States, Canada, Netherlands, Sweden, United Kingdom[26]	Population-based (CRC at various ages) and from clinic-based (Am II)	287 (39)	CRC males: 20% (11%–34%) CRC females: 15% (8%–26%) EC: 15% (6%–35%) LS males: 25% (16%–48%) LS females: 32% (21%–53%)

Abbreviations: Am I, Amsterdam I criteria; Am II, Amsterdam II criteria; CRC, colorectal cancer; EC, endometrial cancer; FH, family history; LS, Lynch syndrome.
[a] Estimates of penetrance likely to be inflated.

have been ascertained through family history of extracolonic malignancies. The investigators reported that the cumulative risk of endometrial cancer was higher in *MSH6* carriers compared with *MLH1* or *MLH2* carriers (27% and 40% respectively).[30] In a study of 70 *MSH6* mutation carriers from 27 families ascertained because of family cancer history meeting the Amsterdam I or II criteria, investigators estimated cumulative colorectal cancer risk in carriers to age 70 of around 80%[31] and reported that the colorectal cancer risk in *MSH6* carriers was lower than that for *MLH1* or *MSH2* carriers.[31] A study of 23 MSH6 mutation carriers of seven population-based probands with double primary colorectal and endometrial cancers.[32] The study reported colorectal cancer risk to age 80 of 61% and endometrial cancer to age 80 of 70.2%.[33] However, because the majority of the germline testing was conducted on affected individuals, this estimate might be biased upwards.[27]

Several studies of *MSH6* mutation penetrance have produced unbiased estimates of risk. In these studies, the mutation carriers were ascertained from families recruited independently of family history or, if they were ascertained because of family history, were appropriately conditioned on the ascertainment.

In a study of mutation-carrying relatives of seven *MSH6* mutation carriers identified from a study of 441 endometrial cancer cases unselected for family history,[18,34] medical record review yielded detailed information for 32 (54%) of the 59 reported cancers and possible precancers in relatives. Investigators tested for the same mutation identified in the proband in the germline of 59 relatives of the probands (21% of all identified relatives), 19 of whom had a confirmed cancer or possible precancer. The investigators' method for estimating penetrance was to divide the number of mutation carriers with a cancer or precancer diagnosis by the total number of carriers identified at each age. After appropriately excluding the probands, as they were ascertained because they had endometrial cancer, investigators estimated that approximately 37% of carriers would develop any cancer or precancerous lesion under the assumption that all cancers/precancers were associated with an *MSH6* mutation.[34] Estimates were only presented for all cancers combined (any cancer) and for males and females combined, and confidence intervals were not provided.

A small meta-analysis of extracted data presented the penetrance estimates based on data from two studies comprising four *MSH6* mutation families from a population-based study of colorectal cancer diagnosed under age 45[35] and six *MSH6* families from the population-based endometrial cancer study described above.[34] The estimated cumulative colorectal cancer risk to age 70 was similar for males and females at approximately 35%.[36] For endometrial cancer, the cumulative risk was approximately 35% to age 70 and 50% to age 80.[36]

The largest study to date drew together an estimated 1043 carriers from 113 families of *MSH6* mutation–carrying probands from five countries ascertained through family cancer clinics and population-based cancer registries.[37] Mutation status, sex, age, and cancer, polypectomy, and hysterectomy histories were sought from 3104 of their relatives. Hazard ratios for cancer risks of carriers compared with those of the general population and age-specific cumulative risks for carriers were estimated using a modified segregation analysis with appropriate conditioning, depending on ascertainment. For carriers, the estimated cumulative risks to age 70 were:

For colorectal cancer:

22% for males
44% to age 80 for males
10% for females

20% to age 80 for females

For endometrial cancer:

26%
44% for age 80

For any Lynch cancer:[37]

24% for males
47% to age 80 for males
40% for females
65% to age 80 for females

PMS2

Previous studies of MMR penetrance have not often included *PMS2* mutation testing and therefore little is known about the cancer risks for *PMS2* mutation carriers. This is primarily due to the difficulty in testing for *PMS2* mutations as discussed above.

There have been multiple reports of individuals with colorectal cancer found to carry two germline *PMS2* mutations (termed *biallelic carriers* in the *PMS2* literature).[5,10,38–41] They typically present with malignancy at a very young age and have gastrointestinal and hematologic malignancies, brain tumors, and neurofibromatosis type I features. There have been only a few reports of individuals with a single PMS2 gene mutations limited to small numbers of probands with deleterious mutations.[30,42]

A study of 33 *PMS2* mutation families ascertained from clinic- and population-based sources that conditioned on ascertainment reported that, compared with the general population, the risk of colorectal cancer for monoallelic carriers was 5.2-fold higher, and the risk of endometrial cancer 7.5-fold higher. In a North America population, this translates to a cumulative cancer risk to age 70 for colorectal cancer of 20% for males and 15% for females; for endometrial cancer of 15%; and for any Lynch syndrome-associated cancer of 25% for males and 32% for females. No elevated risk for non–Lynch syndrome–associated cancers was observed. *PMS2* mutations contribute to Lynch syndrome but the penetrance for monoallelic mutation carriers may be lower than that for the other mismatch repair genes.[26]

SUMMARY

In comparison with the mismatch repair genes *MLH1* and *MSH2*, the genes *MSH6* and *PMS2* are relatively understudied with respect to cancer risk. However, some recent large studies of data combined from several sources, using analytic methods that appropriately condition on the varying methods of ascertainment, are producing reasonably precise estimates, which can be used for risk estimation in patients. To identify modifiers for risk in such carriers, a goal for epidemiologists to improve the health of carriers, such collaborative studies need to continue and expand to include additional mutation carriers in which lifestyle factors and DNA samples are available for analysis.

REFERENCES

1. Kunkel TA, Erie DA. DNA mismatch repair. Annu Rev Biochem 2005;74:681–710.
2. Schofield L, Watson N, Grieu F, et al. Population-based detection of Lynch syndrome in young colorectal cancer patients using microsatellite instability as the initial test. Int J Cancer 2009;124:1097–102.

3. Harfe BD, Jinks-Robertson S. DNA mismatch repair and genetic instability. Annu Rev Genet 2000;34:359–99.
4. Miyaki M, Konishi M, Tanaka K, et al. Germline mutation of MSH6 as the cause of hereditary nonpolyposis colorectal cancer. Nat Genet 1997;17:271–2.
5. Nicolaides NC, Papadopoulos N, Liu B, et al. Mutations of two PMS homologues in hereditary nonpolyposis colon cancer. Nature 1994;371:75–80.
6. Woods MO, Williams P, Careen A, et al. A new variant database for mismatch repair genes associated with Lynch syndrome. Hum Mutat 2007;28:669–73.
7. Nicolaides NC, Carter KC, Shell BK, et al. Genomic organization of the human PMS2 gene family. Genomics 1995;30:195–206.
8. Nicolaides NC, Kinzler KW, Vogelstein B. Analysis of the 5' region of PMS2 reveals heterogeneous transcripts and a novel overlapping gene. Genomics 1995;29:329–34.
9. Nakagawa H, Lockman JC, Frankel WL, et al. Mismatch repair gene PMS2: disease-causing germline mutations are frequent in patients whose tumors stain negative for PMS2 protein, but paralogous genes obscure mutation detection and interpretation. Cancer Res 2004;64:4721–7.
10. De Vos M, Hayward BE, Picton S, et al. Novel PMS2 pseudogenes can conceal recessive mutations causing a distinctive childhood cancer syndrome. Am J Hum Genet 2004;74:954–64.
11. Clendenning M, Hampel H, LaJeunesse J, et al. Long-range PCR facilitates the identification of PMS2-specific mutations. Hum Mutat 2006;27:490–5.
12. Dunlop MG, Farrington SM, Nicholl I, et al. Population carrier frequency of hMSH2 and hMLH1 mutations. Br J Cancer 2000;83:1643–5.
13. Umar A, Boland CR, Terdiman JP, et al. Revised Bethesda Guidelines for hereditary nonpolyposis colorectal cancer (Lynch syndrome) and microsatellite instability. J Natl Cancer Inst 2004;96:261–8.
14. Jass JR. Hereditary non-polyposis colorectal cancer: the rise and fall of a confusing term. World J Gastroenterol 2006;12:4943–50.
15. Hampel H, Frankel WL, Martin E, et al. Feasibility of screening for Lynch syndrome among patients with colorectal cancer. J Clin Oncol 2008;26:5783–8.
16. Hampel H, Stephens JA, Pukkala E, et al. Cancer risk in hereditary nonpolyposis colorectal cancer syndrome: later age of onset. Gastroenterology 2005;129:415–21.
17. Hampel H, Frankel W, Panescu J, et al. Screening for Lynch syndrome (hereditary nonpolyposis colorectal cancer) among endometrial cancer patients. Cancer Res 2006;66:7810–7.
18. Goodfellow PJ, Buttin BM, Herzog TJ, et al. Prevalence of defective DNA mismatch repair and MSH6 mutation in an unselected series of endometrial cancers. Proc Natl Acad Sci U.S.A 2003;100:5908–13.
19. Barnetson RA, Tenesa A, Farrington SM, et al. Identification and survival of carriers of mutations in DNA mismatch-repair genes in colon cancer. N Engl J Med 2006;354:2751–63.
20. Southey MC, Jenkins MA, Mead L, et al. Use of molecular tumor characteristics to prioritize mismatch repair gene testing in early-onset colorectal cancer. J Clin Oncol 2005;23:6524–32.
21. Vasen HF, Watson P, Mecklin JP, et al. New clinical criteria for hereditary nonpolyposis colorectal cancer (HNPCC, Lynch syndrome) proposed by the International Collaborative Group on HNPCC. Gastroenterology 1999;116:1453–6.
22. Jenkins MA, Dowty JG, Hopper JL, et al. Molecular screening of all colorectal tumors diagnosed before age 50 years followed by genetic testing efficiently identifies Lynch syndrome cases. Int J Cancer 2009;124, x–xi.

23. Hampel H, Frankel WL, Martin E, et al. Screening for the Lynch syndrome (hereditary nonpolyposis colorectal cancer). N Engl J Med 2005;352:1851–60.

24. Mead LJ, Jenkins MA, Young J, et al. Microsatellite instability markers for identifying early-onset colorectal cancers caused by germ-line mutations in DNA mismatch repair genes. Clin Cancer Res 2007;13:2865–9.

25. Gill S, Lindor NM, Burgart LJ, et al. Isolated loss of PMS2 expression in colorectal cancers: frequency, patient age, and familial aggregation. Clin Cancer Res 2005; 11:6466–71.

26. Senter L, Clendenning M, Sotamaa K, et al. The clinical phenotype of Lynch syndrome due to germ-line PMS2 mutations. Gastroenterology 2008;135:419–28.

27. Easton DF, Hopper JL, Thomas DC, et al. Breast cancer risks for BRCA1/2 carriers. Science 2004;306:2187–91 [author reply-91].

28. Carayol J, Khlat M, Maccario J, et al. Hereditary non-polyposis colorectal cancer: current risks of colorectal cancer largely overestimated. J Med Genet 2002;39: 335–9.

29. Hendriks YM, Wagner A, Morreau H, et al. Cancer risk in hereditary nonpolyposis colorectal cancer due to MSH6 mutations: impact on counseling and surveillance. Gastroenterology 2004;127:17–25.

30. Hendriks YM, Jagmohan-Changur S, van der Klift HM, et al. Heterozygous mutations in PMS2 cause hereditary nonpolyposis colorectal carcinoma (Lynch syndrome). Gastroenterology 2006;130:312–22.

31. Plaschke J, Engel C, Kruger S, et al. Lower incidence of colorectal cancer and later age of disease onset in 27 families with pathogenic MSH6 germline mutations compared with families with MLH1 or MSH2 mutations: the German Hereditary Nonpolyposis Colorectal Cancer Consortium. J Clin Oncol 2004;22:4486–94.

32. Cederquist K, Emanuelsson M, Goransson I, et al. Mutation analysis of the MLH1, MSH2 and MSH6 genes in patients with double primary cancers of the colorectum and the endometrium: a population-based study in northern Sweden. Int J Cancer 2004;109:370–6.

33. Cederquist K, Emanuelsson M, Wiklund F, et al. Two Swedish founder MSH6 mutations, one nonsense and one missense, conferring high cumulative risk of Lynch syndrome. Clin Genet 2005;68:533–41.

34. Buttin BM, Powell MA, Mutch DG, et al. Penetrance and expressivity of MSH6 germline mutations in seven kindreds not ascertained by family history. Am J Hum Genet 2004;74:1262–9.

35. Jenkins MA, Baglietto L, Dowty JG, et al. Cancer risks for mismatch repair gene mutation carriers: a population-based early onset case-family study. Clin Gastroenterol Hepatol 2006;4:489–98.

36. Chen S, Wang W, Lee S, et al. Prediction of germline mutations and cancer risk in the Lynch syndrome. JAMA 2006;296:1479–87.

37. Baglietto L, Lindor N, Dowty J, et al. Lynch syndrome cancer risks for MSH6 mutation carriers. J Natl Cancer Inst 2009, in press.

38. De Vos M, Hayward BE, Charlton R, et al. PMS2 mutations in childhood cancer. J Natl Cancer Inst 2006;98:358–61.

39. Kruger S, Kinzel M, Walldorf C, et al. Homozygous PMS2 germline mutations in two families with early-onset haematological malignancy, brain tumours, HNPCC-associated tumours, and signs of neurofibromatosis type 1. Eur J Hum Genet 2008;16:62–72.

40. Poley JW, Wagner A, Hoogmans MM, et al. Biallelic germline mutations of mismatch-repair genes: a possible cause for multiple pediatric malignancies. Cancer 2007;109:2349–56.

41. Will O, Carvajal-Carmona LG, Gorman P, et al. Homozygous PMS2 deletion causes a severe colorectal cancer and multiple adenoma phenotype without extraintestinal cancer. Gastroenterology 2007;132:527–30.
42. Worthley DL, Walsh MD, Barker M, et al. Familial mutations in PMS2 can cause autosomal dominant hereditary nonpolyposis colorectal cancer. Gastroenterology 2005;128:1431–6.

Familial Colorectal Cancer Type X: The Other Half of Hereditary Nonpolyposis Colon Cancer Syndrome

Noralane M. Lindor, MD

KEYWORDS

- Cancer • Colorectal • Familial • Hereditary
- Nonpolyposis • HNPCC

The seamstress of Dr A. Warthin predicted that she would die of cancer of either the stomach or the female organs, as that is what happened to her family members, and, indeed, this proved to be true. Dr Warthin, a pathologist at the University of Michigan, began a systematic study of this family, which he called "Family G." He confirmed the cancer diagnoses with histologic findings and published a study on Family G in 1913 (Warthin's contribution reviewed by Merg).[1,2] He subsequently identified other families with similar predisposition to cancer and continued to study, follow, and report on these families into the 1920s. After Warthin, there was general silence in the literature on this subject until a young general internist, Dr Henry Lynch, began to draw attention once again to families such as Family G. He observed that a subset of families with colorectal cancer (CRC) appeared to manifest a highly penetrant, autosomal dominant predisposition to CRC and endometrial cancer. The ages at diagnosis were much lower than those characteristic for those tumors, and the CRCs were located disproportionately in the right colon.[3] He struggled to achieve recognition of this syndrome, as environmental causes of cancer were accepted much more than the possibility that cancer could be hereditary. However, other practitioners gradually began to identify new families that conformed to the Warthin-Lynch observations, and the significance of the family history began to emerge in cancer studies. There were few non-neoplastic or preneoplastic features to distinguish families with Lynch syndrome from sporadic cancer cases, and this clinical entity was given the descriptive name hereditary nonpolyposis colorectal cancer (HNPCC) although there was no formal

Department of Medical Genetics, E7B Mayo Clinic, 200 1st Street SW, Rochester, MN 55905, USA
E-mail address: nlindor@mayo.edu

Surg Oncol Clin N Am 18 (2009) 637–645
doi:10.1016/j.soc.2009.07.003
1055-3207/09/$ – see front matter © 2009 Elsevier Inc. All rights reserved.

surgonc.theclinics.com

definition on how to recognize or diagnose this syndrome. In 1991, after a meeting in Amsterdam, the International Collaborative Group on Hereditary Nonpolyposis Colon Cancer published the Amsterdam I criteria (AC-I) for defining HNPCC.[4] The AC-I are fulfilled if all 4 of the following conditions are met: (1) 3 cases of CRC, in which 2 of the affected individuals are first-degree relatives of the third; (2) CRCs that occur in 2 generations; (3) 1 CRC diagnosed before the age of 50 years; and (4) familial adenomatous polyposis not diagnosed in the family. Creation of a standard definition for HNPCC led rather promptly to identification of germline mutations in DNA mismatch repair (MMR) genes as a cause of Warthin-Lynch syndrome, which came to be called HNPCC by most scientists. Further studies confirmed the dramatically increased risks for cancers of the colorectum and endometrium and also found significantly increased risks for carcinomas of the stomach, small intestine, hepatobiliary tract, kidney, ureter, and ovary. Based on the understanding of the cumulative risks for specific cancers, expert guidelines were provided that stressed cancer surveillance that was to be initiated at very young ages and to be conducted with greater frequency than advised in the general population.[5]

After the discovery of mutations in the DNA MMR genes in families with typical Warthin-Lynch HNPCC, the term "HNPCC" began to be used ambiguously in the medical literature. Some publications defined HNPCC as kindred fulfillment of the Amsterdam criteria (either the original or the revised criteria[4,6]). Some articles stressed that the Amsterdam criteria were designed for research purposes and were overly restrictive for clinical use; nevertheless, they were used clinically. Over time, the term "HNPCC" came to imply the presence of a germline mutation in a DNA MMR gene, especially in laboratory research publications. If all families that fulfilled the Amsterdam criteria actually had germline mutations in DNA MMR genes, this would be nothing more than a semantic problem. However, there was clear evidence that fulfillment of AC-I was not equivalent to having a hereditary DNA MMR gene mutation.[7,8] In a report on 184 probands from 92 Amsterdam criteria–positive families, mutations in MLH1 or MSH2 were found only in 45% of those meeting the criteria.[8] Despite the discovery of MSH6, PMS2, and methods to test for large deletions and the use of tumor microsatellite instability (MSI) testing to help triage cases for germline testing, most studies suggest that only 50% to 60% of families that fulfill the original Amsterdam criteria have a defect in DNA MMR. Note that the Amsterdam II criteria (AC-II), which expand the definition to some of the extracolonic tumors, have a greater sensitivity for underlying hereditary DNA MMR defect.[8]

For that half of families with HNPCC that fulfilled AC-I but did not have DNA MMR gene defects, there was little data on cancer risks or phenotype; there was not even a name to distinguish this group from those with the germline defects—they were all included, by pedigree definition, as HNPCC. But should clinicians counsel that such families need rigorous cancer surveillance and endometrial cancer recommendations driven by the risks associated with hereditary DNA MMR gene mutations? Or might both the magnitude of risks and tumor spectrum be different?

In the largest study to date, the relative risks for cancers were studied in 161 AC-I families from the National Institutes of Health Colon Cancer Family Registry; families with DNA MMR defects were compared with those without DNA MMR defects.[9] MSI in the proband tumor was used to assign MMR status. Ninety families had DNA MMR deficiency, and 71 did not. For purposes of analysis, the Amsterdam-defining "triad" of 3 affected individuals, which always included the proband, was not included in the assessment of cancer risks. The remaining 3422 relatives were either first- or second-degree relatives of a triad member. The incidence of cancer in these relatives was calculated as the ratio of observed-to-expected cases to the number of at-risk person-years (standardized incidence ratio [SIR]). In the families with DNA MMR-deficient tumors, the risk for cancers was statistically significantly elevated for colorectal, endometrial, gastric, small intestine, and kidney or ureter cancers as expected for Lynch syndrome, affirming that the methodology was adequate to detect appropriate information. However, in the 71 families without DNA MMR deficiency, only a twofold-increased risk for CRC was detected (SIR, 2.3; 95% confidence interval, 1.7–3.0), and no other cancer site reached statistical significance for increased risk. An age difference was also apparent: the average age at diagnosis of CRC was higher (61 years) in the families with the tumors with normal DNA MMR compared with families with DNA MMR deficiency (49 years). Based on these data, the authors concluded that families who fulfill the AC-I should not be managed as if they have hereditary DNA MMR defect because the cancer risks are lower and appear to be restricted to CRCs. The term "Lynch syndrome" was used to describe families with hereditary DNA MMR defect, and the term "familial colorectal cancer type X" (FCCTX) was coined to refer to the other HNPCC-like clusters in which no DNA MMR defect could be identified. The word "hereditary" was not included because familial clustering does not prove inheritance, whereas it may imply a Mendelian single-gene–predisposition disorder, which is neither proved nor strongly suspected. "Type X" was chosen because "X" is used as the unknown that needs to be solved in algebraic equations. A call has been made for retirement of the term "HNPCC" because it perpetuates the historical ambiguity of meaning.[10] This study was by no means the first to try to tease apart molecular subsets of high-risk families. **Table 1** summarizes related studies.

An early consideration in Amsterdam criteria–fulfilling families in which no MMR gene mutation could be found was whether the gene mutation was being missed or whether a hereditary MMR gene mutation was creating more subtle disturbances than could be detected with the usual assays for tumor MSI or immunohistochemistry. Renkonen and colleagues[11] tested for allelic messenger RNA (mRNA) expression of *MLH1*, *MSH2*, and *MSH6* by single nucleotide primer extension in 26 pedigree-defined families with HNPCC in which no MMR gene mutation had been detected. They found evidence for undetected germline mutation in an MMR gene in 9 of 11 families that manifest loss of expression of an MMR gene (by tumor immunohistochemistry or MSI) but in none of 15 families with microsatellite-stable (MSS) tumors and normal immunohistochemistry expression of MMR genes. They found evidence for undetected germline MMR mutations in the families with abnormal MMR gene function or expression in the form of unbalanced mRNA expression of *MLH1* in 2 of 11 families and by haplotype analysis in the others. However, in the MSS Amsterdam criteria–fulfilling families, there was no evidence of hypomorphic alleles or undetected mutations in *MLH1*, *MSH2*, or *MSH6*. Schiemann and colleagues[12] extensively tested 25 tumors from 19 Amsterdam criteria–positive cases and 6 Bethesda-guideline cases with reported MSS tumors. They were able to reclassify 2 (8%) of the cases as MSI-high, again suggesting that a missed diagnosis of Lynch syndrome is not a major cause in families with type X colorectal cancer.

To explore whether the tumors of type X cases were similar to or different from those found in Lynch syndrome or in sporadic CRC, Abdel-Rahman and colleagues[13] analyzed the molecular features of the tumors in the pedigree-defined HNPCC group from Finland in which no germline mutations were found or suspected. When 31 tumors from MMR gene–positive families were compared with 18 tumors from gene-negative families, it was concluded that the MMR gene–negative group exhibited a novel molecular pattern characterized by a paucity of changes in the common pathways to colorectal carcinogenesis, distinguishing this group from that with the Lynch syndrome and from that with sporadic CRC. This study supported

Table 1
Overview of studies comparing Amsterdam criteria families with DNA MMR deficiency (Lynch syndrome) and with normal DNA MMR (FCCTX)

	Lynch Families	Type X Families	Comparison between the Lynch and Type X Families
Bisgaard et al[7]	27	12 plus 46 other HNPCC-like	Mutation-negative group less likely to have more than 1 CRC; first cancer more likely to be rectal, less likely to have HNPCC-associated extracolonic tumors; and mean age at diagnosis of first cancer 6 years older
Renkonen et al[11]	11	15[b]	No evidence of MMR gene mutations being missed in type X group, using RNA expression assay
Schiemann et al[12]	NA	19	Type X tumors more likely to be in distal colorectum; 9 years older at diagnosis than MSI-high families
Valle et al[17]	26	38	Type X families 12 years older at diagnosis and CRC more likely to be distal, not mucinous, and probands less likely to have multiple primary tumors
Lindor et al[9]	90	71	Type X had older age and lower risk of diagnosis of CRC; no increased risk for non-CRC tumors
Mueller-Koch et al[15]	25	16	Type X families 11 years older at diagnosis of CRC; only 14% tumors were proximal; fewer synchronous, metachronous, and extracolonic tumors; higher colorectal adenoma to carcinoma ratio suggesting slower progression from precancer to cancer.
Dove-Edwin[16]	26	45[a]	Groups equally likely to develop high-risk adenomas during follow-up, but interval cancers arose only in the Lynch Group. Concluded that surveillance interval can be lengthened in type X
Llor et al[18]	10	15[c]	Type X had more left-sided tumors without tumor-infiltrating lymphocytes; 6 years older at diagnosis; fewer family members with CRC or endometrial cancer

Abbreviation: NA, not applicable, because not described in the article.
[a] Waived the criterion of one person younger than 50 years at diagnosis, so not defined as FCCTX in exactly the same way as in Lindor N, Rabe K, Petersen G, et al. Lower cancer incidence in Amsterdam I criteria families without mismatch repair deficiency: familial colorectal cancer type X. JAMA 2005;293(16):1979–85.
[b] These are HNPCC and HNPCC-like families—proportion of each is unclear.
[c] Used AC-I and AC-II.

the idea of novel predisposition genes and pathways for the families with type X colo-rectal cancer (summarized in **Table 2**).

Sanchez-de-Abajo and colleagues[14] studied 28 tumors from 17 families in Spain that met AC-I or AC-II but in which there was no evidence of MMR defects. RAS, BRAF, and APC somatic mutations were analyzed and expression of methylgua-nine methyltransferase and β-catenin was assessed, and these alterations were correlated with clinical data. This study also supported the concept that families with type X colorectal cancer have distinctive molecular profiles. They reported KRAS mutations in 36% of families, which was similar to reported rates in Lynch syndrome and in sporadic MSS CRCs. Thus the lower rate of KRAS reported by Abdel-Rahman and colleagues[13] was not confirmed. However, they found the KRAS mutations were disproportionately present in codon 12 (83%) compared with equal representation of KRAS mutations between codons 12 and 13 in Lynch syndrome. The KRAS finding was more similar to sporadic CRCs. No association was reported between KRAS mutation and gender or tumor site or stage, but there was a strong association with older age at diagnosis. BRAF mutation, found in 3.6% of families, was not statistically different from Lynch syndrome or sporadic CRCS. Thus the alteration in the RAS/RAF signaling pathway appeared similar between the families with type X cancer and the sporadic MSS cancer, leading the authors to suggest that some families with type X cancer are classified as such because of chance aggregation of sporadic cases. On the other hand, most of the type X CRCs had active Wnt signaling due to either APC or CTNNB1 mutations. The rate of APC mutation was low, about 18%, compared with sporadic MSS CRCs (34%–70%) and similar to Lynch syndrome (21%–27%), and, unexpectedly, small deletions or insertions in repetitive sequences accounted for 70% of mutations, mimicking the profile found in Lynch syndrome. Although the data were not entirely consistent with that reported by Abdel-Rahman and colleagues,[13] sufficient differences were found between the group with type X tumors and that with sporadic CRCs and Lynch syndrome CRCs to be considered distinctive and to warrant additional study.

Several groups have contributed to the clinical understanding of FCCTX. In a study of 41 German families, an older age at CRC diagnosis was noted in FCCTX compared with that in Lynch syndrome (55 vs 41 years); and two-thirds of the tumors were left-sided, the inverse of CRC in Lynch syndrome. The group with Lynch syndrome had more synchronous and metachronous CRCs, but the group with FCCTX had greater adenoma/carcinoma ratio and a tendency toward more adenomas, suggesting a slow-er progression of adenomas to carcinomas.[15] A similar finding was reported in the United Kingdom, based on 97 families with a history of dominant CRC: individuals with Lynch syndrome and FCCTX had equal likelihood of having high-risk adenomas, but only those with Lynch syndrome developed CRC.[16] Among 64 Spanish families that met Amsterdam criteria, 40% had normal DNA MMR in tumor (consistent with other studies) and an older age at CRC diagnosis in the group with FCCTX compared with that in the group with Lynch syndrome (53 vs 41 years); the FCCTX cases were less likely to be in the right colon and had mucinous tumors, and the families had fewer multiple primary tumors.[17] Llor and colleagues[18] studied 100 individuals from 25 Spanish families meeting Amsterdam criteria, of which 40% had normal DNA MMR. Compared with families with known DNA MMR defects, the mean age at diagnosis of CRC in relatives was higher (60 vs 54 years), 89% of tumors were left-sided, and none showed tumor-infiltrating lymphocytes (half of the individuals with Lynch syndrome CRC showed this).[18] **Table 3** compares and contrasts Lynch syndrome with FCCTX, based on the reports from these multiple sources.

Table 2
Molecular characterization of tumors in FCCTX compared with Lynch Syndrome

	Type X, N = 18 Tumors (%)	Lynch, N = 31 Tumors (%)	Sporadic from Literature (%)	P-value for Type X vs Lynch	P-value for Type X vs Sporadic
Nuclear β-catenin	39	81	95	0.005	0.000005
CTNNB1 mutations	0	29	6	0.007	NS
CDX2 alteration: decreased protein	11	6	16	NS	NS
KRAS exon 2 mutations	17	26	30	NS	NS
BRAF V600E	4	0	3	NS	NS
P53 protein stabilization	44	13	52	0.04	NS
TP53 mutation	26	13	52	NS	0.01
Chromosomal instability by CGH	44	Not done	79	—	0.00006

Abbreviations: CGH, comparative genomic hybridization; NS, not significant.
Data from Abdel-Rahman W, Ollikainen M, Kariola R, et al. Comprehensive characterization of HNPCC-related colorectal cancers reveals striking molecular features in families with no germline mismatch repair gene mutations. Oncogene 2005;24(9):1542–51.

Table 3
Contrasting 2 types of families that fulfill the pedigree AC-I

	Lynch Syndrome	FCCTX
Colorectal		
Cancer risk	Very high	Modestly increased
Age of onset	~45 y average	50s–60s
Usual location	Proximal colon	Distal colon
Polyps	Few	More
Malignant transformation	Rapid	Less rapid
Other cancers		
Endometrial risk	Very high risk	Risk not significantly increased
Other cancer sites	Many others	None known
Germline MMR genes	Mutations found	No mutations found
CRC tumor testing	Microsatellite instability	No microsatellite instability (by definition)
CRC tumor staining	Loss of MMR protein expression	Normal expression

Data from Lindor NM. Familial colorectal cancer type X. In: Potter JD, Lindor NM, editors. Genetics of colorectal cancer. Berlin/New York: Springer; 2009.

FCCTX is undoubtedly a heterogenous grouping. It includes some families that have a random aggregation of a common tumor; some families that may be attributable to shared lifestyle factors and/or polygenic predisposition; and some families that likely have a yet-to-be-defined syndrome or undiagnosed single-gene disorders, such as *MYH*-associated polyposis[19] or the MSI-variable families.[20] In a population-based study of 1042 CRC probands with verified family histories, Aaltonen and colleagues[21] explored how much of familial risk is attributable to Lynch syndrome or other known genetic syndromes. When known syndromes were excluded from the analysis, 32% of familial risk remained unaccounted for by the known loci. Genetic modeling of the data did not suggest a better explanation than a simple polygenic model. Studies are now beginning to chip away at the genetic causes of FCCTX.

FCCTX is a diagnosis of exclusion. Care must be exercised in making this diagnosis. Classification depends heavily on tumor MSI results and other laboratory results. One must consider the possibility of a phenocopy within a Lynch syndrome family (ie, a sporadic MSS tumor that arises by chance in a family that actually has Lynch syndrome); one must consider that not all tumors with germline *MSH6* mutations are MSI-high; one must consider laboratory factors, such as the adequacy of the percentage of tumor cells in the MSI-assay and the small but real chance of a falsely normal immunohistochemistry result, if this test is done without MSI testing. In general, the age at diagnosis in the families with FCCTX is greater (see **Table 1**) than that in Lynch syndrome families; and in light of this consistent observation, families with young average age of onset of colorectal tumors or families manifesting other classical Lynch syndrome tumors, such as endometrial cancer, should probably not be categorized as having FCCTX. Cancer-screening recommendations have been suggested for FCCTX, such as offering CRC screening initiated 5 to 10 years before the age of earliest CRC diagnosis in these families, with frequency determined by initial findings but no less often than every 5 years. Aggressive endometrial cancer screening is not supported by current data.[9,16,22] As these guidelines are considerably different and less aggressive than those advised for families with Lynch syndrome, it is essential not to miscategorize families with FCCTX and to continue to reconsider the possibility of a single-gene syndrome, as new disorders are described.

REFERENCES

1. Warthin A. Heredity with reference to carcinoma as shown by the study of the cases examined in the pathological laboratory of the University of Michigan 1895–1913. Arch Intern Med 1913;12:546–55.
2. Merg A, Lynch H, Lynch J, et al. Hereditary colorectal cancer—part II. Curr Probl Surg 2005;42(5):267–333.
3. Lynch H, Shaw M, Magnucoo C, et al. Hereditary factors in cancer: study of two large midwestern kindreds. Arch Intern Med 1966;117:206–12.
4. Vasen H, Mecklin J, Khan P, et al. The International Collaborative Group on Hereditary Non-Polyposis Colorectal Cancer (ICG-HNPCC). Dis Colon Rectum 1991; 334(5):424–5.
5. Burke W, Petersen G, Lynch P, et al. Recommendations for follow-up care of individuals with an inherited predisposition to cancer. I. Hereditary nonpolyposis colon cancer. Cancer Genetics Studies Consortium. JAMA 1997;277(11):915–9.
6. Vasen H, Watson P, Mecklin J, et al. New clinical criteria for hereditary nonpolyposis colorectal cancer (HNPCC, Lynch syndrome) proposed by the International Collaborative group on HNPCC. Gastroenterology 1999;116(6):1453–6.
7. Bisgaard M, Jager A, Myrhoj T, et al. Hereditary non-polyposis colorectal cancer (HNPCC): phenotype-genotype correlation between patients with and without identified mutation. Hum Mutat 2002;20:20–7.
8. Wijnen J, Vasen H, Kahn M, et al. Clinical findings with implications for genetic testing in families with clustering of colorectal cancer. N Engl J Med 1998;339: 511–8.
9. Lindor N, Rabe K, Petersen G, et al. Lower cancer incidence in Amsterdam-I criteria families without mismatch repair deficiency: familial colorectal cancer type X. JAMA 2005;293(16):1979–85.
10. Jass J. Hereditary non-polyposis colorectal cancer: the rise and fall of a confusing term. World J Gastroenterol 2006;12(3):4943–50.
11. Renkonen E, Zhang Y, Lohi H, et al. Altered expression of MLH1, MSH2, and MSH6 in predisposition to hereditary nonpolyposis colorectal cancer. J Clin Oncol 2003;21(19):3629–37.
12. Schiemann U, Muller-Koch Y, Gross M, et al. Extended microsatellite analysis in microsatellite stable, MSH2 and MLH1 mutation-negative HNPCC patients: genetic reclassification and correlation with clinical features. Digestion 2004;69: 166–76.
13. Abdel-Rahman W, Ollikainen M, Kariola R, et al. Comprehensive characterization of HNPCC-related colorectal cancers reveals striking molecular features in families with no germline mismatch repair gene mutations. Oncogene 2005;24(9): 1542–51.
14. Sanchez-de-Abajo A, de la Hoya M, van Puijenbroek M, et al. Molecular analysis of colorectal cancer tumors in patients with mismatch repair-proficient hereditary nonpolyposis colorectal cancer suggests novel carcinogenic pathways. Clin Cancer Res 2007;13(19):5729–35.
15. Mueller-Koch Y, Vogelsang H, Kopp R, et al. Hereditary non-polyposis colorectal cancer: clinical and molecular evidence for a new entity of hereditary colorectal cancer. Gut 2005;54(12):1733–40.

16. Dove-Edwin I, De Jong A, Adams J, et al. Prospective results of surveillance colonoscopy in dominant familial colorectal cancer with and without Lynch syndrome. Gastroenterology 2006;130:1995–2000.
17. Valle L, Perea J, Carbonell P, et al. Clinicopathologic and pedigree differences in Amsterdam-I-positive hereditary nonpolyposis colorectal cancer families according to tumor microsatellite instability status. J Clin Oncol 2007;25(7):781–6.
18. Llor X, Pons E, Xicola R, et al. Differential features of colorectal cancers fulfilling Amsterdam Criteria without involvement of the mutation pathway. Clin Cancer Res 2005;11(20):7304–10.
19. Jenkins M, Croitoru M, Monga N, et al. Risk of colorectal cancer in monoallelic and biallelic carriers of MYH mutations: a population-based case-family study. Cancer Epidemiol Biomarkers Prev 2006;15(2):312–4.
20. Minoo P, Baker K, Goswami R, et al. Extensive DNA methylation in normal colorectal mucosa in hyperplastic polyposis. Gut 2006;55(10):1467–74.
21. Aaltonen L, Johns L, Jarvinen H, et al. Explaining the familial colorectal cancer risk associated with mismatch repair (MMR)-deficient and MMR-stable tumors. Clin Cancer Res 2007;13(1):356–61.
22. Hendriks Y, deJong A, Morreaqu H, et al. Diagnostic approach and management of Lynch syndrome (hereditary nonpolyposis colorectal carcinoma): a guide for clinicians. CA Cancer J Clin 2006;56:213–25.

Less Common Colorectal Cancer Predisposition Syndromes

Thomas J. McGarrity, MD[a,b,]*, Christopher Amos, PhD, FACMG[c,d]

KEYWORDS

- Hamartomatous syndromes • Peutz-Jeghers syndrome
- Juvenile polyposis • Molecular diagnosis
- Clinical management

Familial adenomatous polyposis (FAP), Lynch syndrome (hereditary nonpolyposis colorectal cancer), and MYH-associated polyposis (MAP) are inherited colorectal cancer (CRC) predisposition syndromes that taken together account for approximately 5% of the annual incidence of CRC in the United States.[1–4] The far less common hamartomatous polyposis syndromes are a heterogeneous group of inherited CRC conditions accounting for less than 1% of the CRC incidence.[5,6] Historically, individuals with hamartomatous polyposis syndromes were classified by their unique phenotypic features and "classic" polyp histology. In the clinical setting, features of the hamartomatous syndromes are often overlapping leading to challenging diagnostic and management decisions. Hyperplastic polyposis (HP) syndrome is a rare, relatively newly described entity, and affected individuals have an increased risk of CRC.[7–9] Multiple polyp types are characteristic of individuals with HP and hamartomatous polyposis syndrome.[4–10] Misclassification of polyp histopathology has delayed in part the recognition of HP and the sessile serrated neoplasia CRC pathway.[8,10–19]

Recently, predictive gene testing identifying the molecular mutations responsible for the hamartomatous syndromes has provided diagnostic clarity and improved clinical

[a] Department of Medicine, Penn State Hershey Medical Center, 500 University Drive, H045, Hershey, PA 17033–0850, USA
[b] Division of Gastroenterology and Hepatology, Penn State Hershey Medical Center, 500 University Drive, H045, Hershey, PA 17033–0850, USA
[c] Section of Informatics, Department of Epidemiology, 3240 University of Texas, MD Anderson Cancer Center, 1155 Pressler Street, Houston, TX 77039–4009, USA
[d] Section of Computational and Genetic Epidemiology, University of Texas, MD Anderson Cancer Center, Houston, TX, USA
* Corresponding author. Division of Gastroenterology and Hepatology, Penn State Hershey Medical Center, 500 University Drive, H045, Hershey, PA 17033–0850.
E-mail address: tmcgarrity@hmc.psu.edu (T.J. McGarrity).

Surg Oncol Clin N Am 18 (2009) 647–661
doi:10.1016/j.soc.2009.07.005
1055-3207/09/$ – see front matter. Published by Elsevier Inc.

surgonc.theclinics.com

management by allowing earlier and more targeted interventions. Proper identification and characterization of these less common syndromes demands a strong collaborative effort among clinicians, genetic counselors, and pathologists. The central role for the pathologist was highlighted in a recent report by Sweet and colleagues[10] of 49 patients with unexplained polyposis.[10] Central pathology review of 23 patients with synchronous hyperplastic and adenomatous polyps increased the prevalence of sessile serrated adenomas from 13% to 57%.[10] In these rare syndromes, the genetic counselor plays a pivotal vital role in elucidating the complete family medical history, directing a strategy for germline mutation testing, and educating and counseling the patient and at-risk family members about the ramifications of predictive gene testing (discussed elsewhere in this issue).[1–3,5,20–23] The total cancer burden in the hamartomatous polyposis syndromes is significant, including both intestinal and extraintestinal malignancies. Reclassification of these syndromes based on a molecular diagnosis will improve disease risk stratification and the organ-specific risk of cancer including CRC. In addition to uncovering the pathogenesis of cancer in these individuals, molecular understanding of these less common CRC predisposition syndromes will likely yield insights into the genesis of cancer in general. Specifically, as FAP syndrome and the Lynch syndrome exemplify two distinct pathways to CRC, HP may represent the familial form of a third CRC pathway, the serrated neoplasia pathway, and understanding the molecular basis of juvenile polyposis (JP) and Peutz-Jeghers syndrome (PJS) has led to new insights into the development of many epithelial cancers.

HP SYNDROME

Historically, the adenoma was considered the sole macroscopic CRC precursor. The risk of malignant transformation of hyperplastic polyps was believed to be nil. More recently, this long held tenet has been challenged. Hereditary polyposis syndrome was initially described in the late 1970s.[7,11,12] The familial clustering of HP suggests a genetic origin.[4,7–10,18,24,25] Clinically, HP syndrome should be suspected in an individual with multiple large colonic hyperplastic polyps. The clinical criteria for HP are listed in **Box 1**.[9]

In some publications, the criteria for HP have been modified to include individuals with more than 20 hyperplastic polyps.[8]

The clinical and histologic picture of HP is evolving and may involve two phenotypes including a pancolonic distribution of hyperplastic polyps and a more restricted polyposis proximal to the sigmoid colon. From the University of Utah, 15 patients with HP underwent 65 colonoscopies with an average of 15 polypectomies per procedure. Although hyperplastic polyps were evenly distributed throughout the large bowel, hyperplastic polyps greater than 1 cm predominated in the proximal colon (38 proximal versus 13 distal).[26]

Multiple synchronous colon polyp histology typifies HP. A Swedish study of 10 HP patients noted that eight HP individuals had additional serrated adenomas, and seven

---

Box 1
World Health Organization international diagnostic criterion of HP

1. At least five histologically diagnosed hyperplastic polyps proximal to the sigmoid colon of which two are greater than 10 mm in diameter

2. Any number of hyperplastic polyps occurring proximal to the sigmoid colon in an individual who has a first-degree relative with HP

3. Greater than 30 hyperplastic polyps but distributed throughout the colon

were diagnosed with typical tubulovillous or villous adenomas.[27] In the work of Chow and colleagues,[25] 84% of HP patients had synchronous mixed polyp histology. The need for an expert gastrointestinal pathologist was underscored in the study by Sweet and colleagues[10] In another study, a second look by an expert pathologist reclassified 18% of hyperplastic polyps as sessile serrated adenomas.[13]

Although not appreciated initially, the CRC risk of HP is now recognized to be significant.[24–28] Williams and colleagues[29] followed seven HP patients up to 13 years and none developed CRC. In contrast, 7 of 10 HP patients reported from Sweden were diagnosed with CRC with a mean age of 62 years (range, 39–77 years).[27] The largest series of HP syndrome (N = 38) was reported by Chow and colleagues in 2006.[25] Adenomas were noted in 26% of individuals, and 50% of patients had a first-degree relative with CRC. Ten of the 38 patients developed CRC with a median and mean age of 45 and 49 years, respectively. An additional three required colon resection for diffuse polyposis. Cancers were evenly distributed throughout the large bowel, although the larger hyperplastic polyps (>10 mm) tended to be proximal to the sigmoid colon. Furthermore, Rubio and colleagues[27] collected the world literature of HP and 67 (51%) of 131 HP patients had developed CRC.

Endoscopic detection and removal of hyperplastic polyps can be problematic because the polyps tend to be flatter than typical adenomas and may escape recognition at the time of colonoscopies. CRC arising in areas of prior hyperplastic polypectomy sites, especially in the proximal colon, have been reported.[19,30–40]

Chromoendoscopy with indigo carmine is a valuable technique, especially in the proximal colon, to identify these lesions.[19,32,41–43] All polyps greater than 5 mm from the proximal colon should be removed because three quarters of these may be sessile serrated adenomas with a greater predilection to cancer development.[19] Careful inspection of colonic folds and a slow withdrawal time are paramount for high-quality colonoscopic examination for polyp detection.[35,44] Newer endoscopic technologies including narrow band and confocal microscopy imaging may offer additional advantages for hyperplastic polyp detection.[32,35,41]

Endoscopic mucosal resection with the injection of saline into the submucosal space to elevate the lesion off the muscularis propria allows for safer resection of these minimally elevated flat lesions.[19,32,41] An endoscopic piecemeal removal of a large flat polyp should be followed up in 3 to 6 months to ensure complete polyp removal. India ink tattoo is helpful for site identification. After all polyps have been removed, individuals should be enrolled in a colonoscopic surveillance program. Colonoscopic surveillance every 1 to 3 years based on the polyp size, number, and histology has been recommended.[19,25] Some experts have suggested a more aggressive colonoscopic surveillance strategy. For a young individual who presents initially with HP and a synchronous cancer, total colectomy with ileorectal anastomosis is recommended. This decreases the area at risk for subsequent cancer development and simplifies endoscopic surveillance. Additional HP individuals present with multiple large right-sided hyperplastic polyps. The decision to remove these endoscopically versus colectomy with ileorectal anastomosis needs to be individualized. First-degree relatives should be counseled and offered surveillance colonoscopy beginning 10 years younger than the age of the index case of cancer in the family.[8,24,25]

GENETICS OF HP

There are increasing data indicating that HP demonstrates an alternative pathway to CRC. As FAP and Lynch syndrome represents the inherited conditions representative of the chromosome instability and microsatellite instability CRC pathways, respectively, HP may be the hereditary form of the serrated adenoma pathway to CRC. Dysplastic areas of hyperplastic polyps were found to show high-frequency microsatellite instability.[15,16] Microsatellite instability, characteristic of Lynch syndrome–associated CRC, also occurs in 15% of sporadic CRCs, primarily from the proximal colon.[45] APC loss and KRAS do not occur in non-Lynch sporadic high-frequency microsatellite instability tumors. In contrast, APC loss and KRAS do occur frequently in Lynch syndrome–associated colorectal tumors.[46]

Islands of CpG dinucleotide repeats present in the 5' promoter regions of genes are typically unmethylated. DNA methylation is a common epigenetic mechanism for gene silencing. Hypermethylation of the promoter region of the mismatch repair gene, MLH-1, (so-called "CpG island methylator phenotype") may be the molecular pathway responsible for the progression of hyperplastic polyps to sessile serrated adenomas to colon cancer.[15–19,46] Mutations in the BRAF oncogene are common in CRC arising from sessile serrated adenomas but not in Lynch syndrome–associated CRC, whereas KRAS and APC gene mutations are common.[46,47] It has been estimated that 20% of all CRCs may originate from this pathway.[17]

The genetic basis of HP-associated CRC is evolving. No germline mutation for HP has yet been determined. Some pedigrees are consistent with autosomal-dominant inheritance pattern. In the report by Chow and colleagues[25] one individual was found to have a biallelic MYH mutation. The authors suggested testing for MYH mutations in patients with HP and concomitant adenomas. In the report by Sweet and colleagues[10] two individuals had PTEN mutations, although the phenotypes were not diagnostic for Cowden disease. Testing of tumor tissue for BRAF and KRAS may improve the classification and diagnosis of HP.[18,47] In one study, a BRAF mutation was present in 42% of 40 tumors with a loss of the mismatch repair gene MLH-1 by immunohistochemistry but in none of 28 tumors with loss of MLH-2 expression.[47]

HAMARTOMATOUS POLYPOSIS SYNDROME

The hamartomatous polyposis syndromes occur significantly less often than the adenomatous polyposis syndromes, FAP, MAP, and Lynch syndrome. The hamartomatous polyposis syndromes are characterized by an overgrowth of cells native to the area in which they normally occur.[6] All are autosomal-dominantly inherited conditions. Common to their adenomatous polyposis counterparts, a family history is often lacking and de novo mutations occur at a high rate. There is a marked phenotypic overlap of these syndromes and a molecular diagnosis has become the gold standard.[46] Despite these advances, however, a definable germline mutation genetic alteration is found in only 50% of individuals tested. There is a pressing need for strong collaboration among clinicians, genetic counselors, and pathologists. Affected and at-risk individuals are at very high risk for intestinal and extraintestinal malignancies. The genetic counselor is critical for the careful gathering of the family history and pathologic material and is pivotal for generating a genetic differential diagnosis and prioritizing the genetic germline testing.[3,20–23] There are classic pathologic features of the hamartomatous polyps in these syndromes. There is significant overlap and an expert gastrointestinal pathologist is critical for accurate diagnosis and subsequent patient management decisions.

The phosphatase and tensin homolog (PTEN) hamartoma syndrome includes Cowden disease and Bannayan-Riley-Ruvalcaba syndrome.[1,2,6] Cowden disease, also known as the "multiple hamartoma syndrome," is characterized by ectodermal, mesodermal, and endodermal hamartomas that are most pronounced in skin, breast, thyroid, and intestine. In general, an increased risk for gastrointestinal malignancy has not been shown.[48–54] One study showed, however, that 10% of 93 Cowden disease patients in a Japanese registry had colon cancer.[55] Although there is little or no increased risk for intestinal cancers, individuals with PTEN mutations have elevated risk for breast, follicular thyroid, and endometrial cancers.[52,53] Diagnostic criteria for PTEN-hamartoma syndromes are well established.[54]

JP SYNDROME

JP is the most common hamartomatous syndrome occurring in approximately 1 per 100,000 births. Hamartomatous polyps of JP affect primarily the colon but also the upper gastrointestinal tract.[6,56,57] It is important to distinguish JP from sporadic juvenile polyps, which can occur in up to 2% of the pediatric population.[6] Only 50% of patients with syndromic JP, however, have a family history of the disorder.

The clinical diagnosis of JP is made when any of the three criteria are met (**Box 2**)[57]: (1) multiple[3–10] colonic hamartomatous polyps, (2) any number of hamartomatous polyps in a patient with a family history of JP, or (3) extracolonic hamartomatous polyps.

Typically, JP polyps are smooth, round sessile lesions but larger polyps are pedunculated. These polyps are friable and frequently undergo autoamputation. They often present with frank hematochezia or occult anemia. Histologically, they are multilobulated polyps with cystically dilated glands within an inflamed stroma, which lacks the prominent smooth muscle bundles seen in classic Peutz-Jeghers polyps. CRC is believed to arise from foci of dysplasia or through concomitant adenomatous polyps.[58–60]

The CRC risk in JP is significant[1,58–63] and has been noted in 9% to 68% of JP patients with a mean age at diagnosis of 34 years. A 17% to 22% risk of CRC by age 35 increases to 68% by age 60 years.[56] In the Hopkins polyposis registry, the risk assessment for CRC in JP showed a relative risk of 34 compared with the United States population with a cumulative lifetime risk of 39%.[58] The mean age of diagnosis of CRC in the JP Hopkins registry was 44 years. In JP patients with gastric polyps, the incidence of gastric adenocarcinoma was 21%.[56]

This marked increased risk for CRC in JP syndrome leads to endorsement of screening and surveillance.[1,6,56–65] Screening of at-risk individuals with molecular testing is preferred. If not possible, screening colonoscopy every 3 years is recommended beginning in the teenage years or at the onset of symptoms. Affected individuals should have biannual colonoscopy beginning at age 15 years. Surveillance colonoscopy is performed based on individual polyp burden. Diffuse polyposis may require colectomy. The development of invasive CRC mandates definitive surgery with or without ileorectal anastomosis depending on the degree of rectal involvement.

Box 2
Jass criteria for JP

Syndrome[57]

- ≥5 hamartomatous polyps in the colorectum[a]
- Any hamartomatous polyps in the colorectum in a patient with a positive family history of JP
- Any hamartomatous polyps in the stomach or small intestine[a]

[a] In the absence of clinical findings consistent with other hamartomatous polyposis syndromes (eg, BRRS and Cowden's Syndrome).

Starting in the teenage years, screening for gastric and duodenal cancer by upper endoscopy every 2 to 3 years, although not universally recommended, is a reasonable recommendation.[1,8,56,57,64,65]

Genetics of JP

The development of JP has been linked to abnormalities in transforming growth factor-β, an important signal transduction pathway.[57,66,67] Genetic alterations in *SMAD4* located on chromosome 18, *BMPR1A* (bone, morphogenic, protein receptor 1A), chromosome 10, and *ENG* (endoglin), an accessory TGF-β receptor, are found in approximately 50% of affected JP syndrome individuals.[66,68–70] In mice, *BMPR1A* inactivation leads to the development of intestinal polyposis.[67] Endoglin mutations are responsible for hereditary hemorrhagic telangiectasia (Osler-Weber-Rendu disease), which does not confer substantial risk for polyposis.[71] Some individuals with *SMAD4* mutations show a combined phenotype of hemorrhagic telangiectasia and JP, however, and are at increased risk for arteriovascular malformations.[10,72] A rare subset of JP patients with large deletions of *BMPR1A* and *PTEN* show a contiguous gene syndrome comprising early manifestations of severe generalized polyposis of infancy, typically occurring by age 2.[73–76] The course of disease in these children is marked by recurrent gastrointestinal bleeding, obstruction, secretory diarrhea, and a limited lifespan. There are data to suggest that mutations in BMPs do not decrease CRC risk. Mutations in *SMAD4* have been associated with increased risk for both CRC and gastric cancer.[73–77] Aside from missense and nonsense mutations, some patients with JP syndrome have been found to have large deletions of either *SMAD4* or *BMPR1A*, detectable by the multiplex ligation-dependent probe assay.[73,78,79]

PEUTZ-JEGHERS SYNDROME

In 1921, Dr. Jan Peutz reported a 15-year-old boy with distinctive facial macules and intestinal polyposis causing intussusception. Three additional family members had intestinal polyposis and facial hyperpigmentation.[80] Jeghers and coworkers[81] further described the familial association of intestinal polyposis and hyperpigmented macule of the face, lips, digits, and mucous membranes. Polyps in PJS can be seen throughout the gastrointestinal tract but are ubiquitous in the jejunum. Peutz-Jeghers polyps are characterized by a smooth muscle core, which is tightly adherent to the bowel wall. PJS polyps undergo autoamputation less commonly than in JP, and are more like to cause abdominal pain, obstruction, and intussusception. The classic PJS polyp with arborizing smooth muscle bands is seen in the small bowel, whereas gastric and colonic PJS hamartomas contains less muscle and can demonstrate cystically dilated glands and inflammation reminiscent of JP polyps, and adenomatous polyps are also common in the colon. Polyps in PJS have also been found in the naris, gallbladder, urogenital, and respiratory tracts. In a large series of 82 PJS patients, 96% had small bowel polyps, 27% had colorectal polyps, and 24% had stomach polyps.[82] PJS polyposis occurs early in life. The median time to presentation of polyps is approximately 11 years, over one third of patients develop symptoms within the first decade of life, and 60% before age 20 years.[82,83]

The mucocutaneous hyperpigmentation is seen in up to 95% of affected individuals, and is characterized by small (1–5 mm) dark blue to dark brown macules around the mouth, eyes, nostrils, perianal area, and buccal membranes and often precedes the gastrointestinal manifestations. Hyperpigmented macules on the digits are common. It is important to clinically recognize that the cutaneous pigmented lesions may fade in puberty and adulthood. A similar benign form of pigmentation without polyposis termed the "Laugier-Hunziker syndrome" needs to be considered.

The PJS hamartoma with the characterizing arborising pattern of overgrowth in the muscularis mucosa predispose these lesions to intestinal obstruction and intussusception. This results in a need for repeated surgeries and bowel loss often leading to short bowel syndrome and malabsorption. A proactive approach of prophylactic endoscopic polypectomy has been advocated, which may decrease the need for emergency surgery and limits the surgical loss of intestine that can be required to correct intussusceptions.

Routine endoscopy (**Table 1**) with small bowel enteroscopy and colonoscopy with polypectomy have become the standard recommendations.[64,65,84,85] Video wireless capsule endoscopy has been shown to give a more accurate visualization of the small intestine in polyposis syndromes and if available, has supplanted barium contrast studies of the small bowel.[86,87] Double-balloon enteroscopy is a newer technique where one balloon is attached to the tip of a 200-cm working length endoscope, and the second balloon is attached to the distal end of a soft overtube. With a series of maneuvers, the more distal small bowel can be visualized.[88,89] Double-balloon enteroscopy allows for polypectomy (**Fig. 1**). In one study of nine polyposis patients, double-balloon endoscopy detected a larger number of polyps than capsule endoscopy. Furthermore, double-balloon enteroscopy detected polyps in three patients with negative capsule endoscopy readings.[88]

At endoscopy, all polyps greater than 1 cm in reach of the endoscope should be removed. Surgery with intraoperative endoscopy to remove all polyps of significant size, the so called "clean sweep," is recommended by some experts and may decrease the need for recurrent emergent small bowel surgery.[90] Given the widespread geography of PJS polyps within the gastrointestinal tract, conservative surgery to decrease bowel loss is recommended.

Table 1
Surveillance recommendations for PJS Individual

Screened Cancer	Age to Begin Screening (Yrs)	Interval (Yrs)	Diagnostic Tests
Colon	18	2–3	Colonoscopy
Proximal GI Tract	8	2–3	Upper endoscopy/ enteroscopy and small bowel[a,b] series
Pancreas	25–30	1–2	Endoscopic ultrasound
Breast	25	1	MRI[c]/Mammography
Uterus/Cervix	21	1	Pelvic exam with pap smear
Ovaries	25	1	Transvaginal ultrasound and serum CA-125
Testicles	Birth	1	Physical examination and ultrasound if clinically indicated

[a] Depending on local availability, capsule endoscopy may replace small bowel series.
[b] Consider intraoperative endoscopy to remove polyps >1.5 cm. depending on local availability;- double-balloon enteroscopy might replace the need for laparotomy and intraoperative endoscopy.
[c] MRI more sensitive in high risk groups and younger patients.

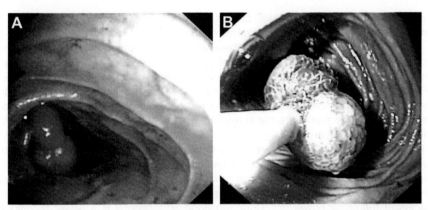

Fig. 1. A jejunal polyp in an 18-year-old woman with Peutz-Jeghers syndrome detected by video capsule endoscopy but beyond the reach of conventional small bowel enteroscopy. The polyp was detected (*A*) and removed (*B*) by double-balloon enteroscopy. (*Courtesy of Dr. Nake Pooran, Gastroenterology Division, Penn State Hershey Medical Center, Hershey, PA.*)

With advancing age, intestinal cancer becomes the major clinical concern in individuals with PJS.[84,91–100] The coexistence of adenomatous tissue within Peutz-Jeghers hamartomas of stomach, small bowel, and colorectum has been demonstrated and has been termed the "hamartoma-adenoma-carcinoma sequence."[101–103] PJS patients may also have increased risk of adenomas. The cancer burden of PJS including intestinal and extraintestinal malignancies is high. Gallione and colleagues has shown cumulative risk for all cancers of 93% with a marked increased relative rate for breast, colon, pancreatic, stomach, and ovarian cancer.[72] The lifetime risk of breast cancer for female patients is over 50%,[96] which approaches the magnitude noted in the hereditary breast cancer predisposition syndromes BRCA1 and BRCA2. In addition, distinctive nonneoplastic and neoplastic genital tract tumors in male and female patients occur. Female PJS patients are at risk for ovarian sex cord tumors with annular tubules in addition to mucinous tumors of the ovary and fallopian tubes, and a well-differentiated adenoma-carcinoma of the uterine cervix termed "adenoma malignum." Males with PJS are at risk for developing testicular tumors classified as large cell calcifying Sertoli cell tumors, and testicular tumors resembling sex cord tumors with annular tubules. Males with these tumors present with rapid growth, advanced for age, and gynecomastia caused by increased aromatase activity and estrogen products.[1–4,98,99] If nonmalignant, small testicular tumors can initially be managed using aromatase inhibitors.

In 240 PJS patients with documented germline mutations, the risk of cancer at age 20, 30, 40, 50, 60, and 70 years was 1%, 3%, 19%, 13%, 63%, and 81%, respectively.[99] In a 78-year-old follow-up of the original family described by Peutz from the Hague, seven cancers were diagnosed in 22 affected individuals. Five of the seven tumors occurred in the gastrointestinal tract, and three were CRCs with a mean age of cancer diagnosis of 50 years.[94] In a meta-analysis of 210 PJS patients, the relative risk for large bowel cancer was 98 compared with the general population.[95] In the series by Giardiello and colleagues[92] the risk of developing CRC by age 65 years was 39%. In a review by Spigelman and colleagues[93] three fourths of the gastrointestinal malignancies occurred before the age of 50 years. These studies may suffer from biases inherent in registry-based cohort studies, in which the most seriously affected individuals are retained by the registry. Boardman and colleagues,[104] however, identified and contacted all patients seen at the Mayo Clinic in a systematic fashion and observed a 148-fold increased risk for all cancers in women with a 20-fold higher breast cancer compared with expected frequencies from the United States population and a sixfold increased risk for cancer in men, further excess risk for cancer that occurs in PJS.

At risk first-degree relatives of PJS patients should undergo an annual history and physical examination with specific evaluation for characteristic mucocutaneous pigmentation, precocious puberty, and testicular tumors. Because of the early onset of symptoms in PJS, at-risk children should be offered predictive gene testing for mutations in the STK11 gene. Testing of young at-risk individuals is justified in that in some series, 30% of PJS patients by age 10 undergo emergent laparotomy for small bowel obstruction.[84] Identifying an STK11 mutation in an affected family member has major implications for at-risk family members. In this instance, a person with a negative mutation test can avoid the vigorous surveillance guidelines. As for the other hamartomatous polyposis syndromes, if the gene testing is uninformative, at-risk individuals with characteristic mucocutaneous pigmentation should follow the surveillance guidelines as stated.

Genetics

The genetic basis of PJS was established by the identification of a novel human serine-threonine kinase gene (STK11, also sometimes referred to as LKB1).[105,106] All mutations found in an early study of 23 familial and two sporadic cases of PJS were predicted to lead to synthesis of a truncated protein predicted to result in loss of function of the kinase domain and activity.[105] PJS is the first cancer predisposition syndrome that is the result of loss of catalytic activity of a serine-threonine kinase. The effect of haploinsufficiency versus loss of function from both alleles and polyp formation has yet to be resolved. In a mouse model, heterozygosity for LKB1 mutations suggesting haploinsufficiency was sufficient to cause polyp formation and growth.[107] More recent kindred analysis demonstrated a decrease of prevalence of LKB1 mutations compared with earlier studies suggesting another susceptibility locus for PJS. STK11 mutations are present in approximately 50% to 90% of individuals with PJS phenotype depending on the series. Aside from truncating mutations, larger deletions including deletions of the entire gene and missense mutations have all been shown to cause PJS. Relatively few studies have characterized genotype phenotype correlations of STK11 and PJS. Missense mutations correlated with the later onset of gastrointestinal symptoms with decrease incidence of intussusception compared with truncating mutations or compared with cases without detectable mutations.[83]

SUMMARY

A variety of syndromes confer increased risk for intestinal polyp development, outside the more commonly occurring syndromes of FAP, MAP, and hereditary nonpolyposis colorectal cancer. Each of these uncommon syndromes predispose to pathognomonic histologies that are uncommonly observed. Accurate diagnosis of these syndromes is contingent on higher-level pathology review; evaluation of signs and symptoms beyond sole consideration of the polyps; and collection of a detailed family history, including ages at onset of polypoid development in first-degree relatives, a family history of cancers, and signs and symptoms in the relatives. When a genetic mutation can be identified in the proband, the management of intestinal and extraintestinal cancer screening can be more appropriately tailored. In particular, in the absence of a positive test result in the proband, at-risk first-degree relatives are advised to undergo routine screening. If the proband tests positive for a mutation, then relatives testing negative for mutations are not at elevated risk for polyp or cancer development and can avoid routine screenings.

ACKNOWLEDGMENT

The author expresses gratitude to Beverly Bell for her superb secretarial assistance.

REFERENCES

1. Burt R, Neklason DW. Genotic testing for inherited colon cancer. Gastroenterology 2005;128:1696–716.
2. Doxey BW, Kuwada SK, Burt RW. Inherited polyposis syndrome: molecular mechanism, clinicopathology, and genetic testing. Clin Gastroenterol Hepatol 2005;3:633–41.
3. Lynch HT, Lynch JF, Lynch PM, et al. Hereditary colorectal cancer syndrome: molecular genetics, genetic counseling, diagnosis and management. Fam Cancer 2008;7:27–9.
4. Rustgi AK. The genetics of hereditary colon cancer. Genes Dev 2007;24: 2525–38.
5. Carethers JM. Unwinding the heterogeneous nature of hamartomatous polyposis syndromes. JAMA 2005;294:2498–500.
6. Schreibman IR, Baker M, Amos C, et al. The hamartomotous polyposis syndrome: a clinical and molecular review. Am J Gastroenterol 2005;100: 476–90.
7. Cooke SA. Polyposis coli: the clinical spectrum in adults. S Afr Med J 1978;53: 454–7.
8. Rashid A, Houlihan PS, Booker S, et al. Phenotypic and molecular characteristics of hyperplastic polyposis. Gastroenterology 2000;119:323–32.
9. Burt RW, Jass JR. Hyperplastic polyposis. In: Hamilton SR, Aaltonen LA, editors. World Health Organization classification of tumours. Pathology and genetics. Tumours of the digestive system. Lyon: IARC Press; 2000. p. 135–6.
10. Sweet K, Willis J, Zhou X-P, et al. Molecular classification of patients with unexplained hamartomatous and hyperplastic polyposis. JAMA 2005;294:2465–73.
11. Spjut H, Estrada R. The significance of epithelial polyps of the large bowel. Pathol Annu 1977;12:147–70.
12. Cooper HS, Patchefsky AS, Marks G. Adenomatous and carcinomatous changes within hyperplastic colonic epithelium. Dis Colon Rectum 1979;22: 152–6.
13. Torlakovic E, Snover DC. Serrated adenomatous polyposis in humans. Gastroenterology 1996;110:748–55.
14. Beusnel C, Le Berre N, Pagenault M, et al. Giant hyperplastic polyposis with adenomatous tissue. Gastroenterol Clin Biol 1996;20:294–7.
15. Jass JR, Lino H, Ruszkiewicz A, et al. Neoplastic progression occurs through mutator pathways in hyperplastic polyposis of the colorectum. Gut 2000;47: 43–9.
16. Jass JR, Whitehall V, Young J, et al. Emerging concepts in colorectal neoplasia. Gastroenterology 2002;123:862–76.
17. Park S-J, Rashid A, Lee J-H, et al. Frequent CpG island methylation in serrated adenomas of the colorectum. Am J Pathol 2003;162:815–22.

18. Carvajal-Carmona LG, Howarth KM, Lockett M, et al. Molecular classification and genetic pathways in hyperplastic polyposis syndrome. J Pathol 2007;212: 379–85.
19. East JE, Saunders BP, Jass JR. Sporadic and syndronic hyperplastic polyps and serrated adenomas of the colon; classification molecular genetics, natural history and clinical management. Gastroenterol Clin North Am 2008;37:25–46.
20. Petersen GM, Brensinger JD, Johnson KA, et al. Genetic testing and counseling for hereditary forms of colorectal cancer. Cancer 1999;86:2540–50.
21. Guttmacher AE, Collins FS, Carmona RH. The family history: more important than ever. N Engl J Med 2004;351:2333–6.
22. Rubinstein WS, Weissman SM. Managing hereditary gastrointestinal cancer syndromes: the partnership between genetic counselors and gastroenterologists. Nat Clin Proc Gastroenterology Hepatol 2008;5:569–82.
23. Lynch HT, Boland CR, Rodriques-Bigas MA, et al. Who should be sent for genetic testing in hereditary colorectal causes syndromes? J Clin Oncol 2007; 25:3534–42.
24. Lage P, Cravo M, Sousa R, et al. Management of Portuguese patients with hyperplastic polyposis and screening of at-risk first-degree relatives: a contribution for future guidelines based on a clinical study. Am J Gastroenterol 2004;99: 1779–84.
25. Chow E, Lipton L, Lynch E, et al. Hyperplastic polyposis syndrome: phenotypic presentations and the role of MBD4 and MYH. Gastroenterology 2006;131:30–9.
26. Ferrandez A, Samowitz W, DiSario J, et al. Phenotypic characteristics and risk of cancer development in hyperplastic polyposis: case series and literature review. Am J Gastroenterol 2004;99:2012–8.
27. Rubio CA, Stemme S, Jaramillo E, et al. Hyperplastic polyposis coli syndrome and colorectal carcinoma. Endoscopy 2006;38:266–70.
28. Hyman NH, Anderson P, Blasyk H. Hyperplastic polyposis and the risk of colorectal cancer. Dis Colon Rectum 2004;47:2101–4.
29. Williams GT, Arthur JF, Bussey HJ, et al. Hyperplastic-adenomatous polyposis syndrome. J Am Coll Surg 1999;188:503–7.
30. Koide N, Saito Y, Fujii T, et al. A case of hyperplastic polyposis of the colon with adenocarcinomas in hyperplastic polyps after long-term follow-up. Endoscopy 2002;34:499–502.
31. Rex DK, Ulbright TM. Step section histology of proximal colon polyps that appear hyperplastic by endoscopy. Am J Gastroenterol 2002;97:1530–4.
32. Soetikno RM, Kaltenbach T, Rouse RV, et al. Prevalence of nonpolypoid (flat and depressed) colorectal neoplasms in asymptomatic and symptomatic adults. JAMA 2008;299:1027–35.
33. Lieberman D, Nadel M, Smith R, et al. Standardized colonoscopy reporting and data system (CO-RADS): report of the Quality Assurance Task Group of the National Colorectal Cancer Roundtable. Gastrointest Endosc 2007;65:757–66.
34. Goldstein NS, Shanot P, Odish E. Hyperplastic-like colon polyps that preceded microsatellite-unstable adenocarcinomas. Am J Clin Pathol 2003;119:778–96.
35. Rex DK. Maximizing detection of adenomas and cancers during colonoscopy. Am J Gastroenterol 2006;101:2866–77.
36. Jass JR. Hyperplastic-like polyps as precursors of microsatellite-unstable colorectal cancer. Am J Clin Pathol 2003;119:773–5.
37. O'Brien MJ, Yang S, Clebanoff JL, et al. Hyperplastic (serrated) polyps of the colorectum: relationship of CpG island methylator phenotype and K-ras mutation to location and histologic subtype. Am J Surg Pathol 2004;28:423–34.

38. Sheridan TB, Fenton H, Lewis MT, et al. Sessile serrated adenomas with low-and high-grade dysplasia and early carcinomas: an immunohistochemical study of serrated lesions "caught in the act". Am J Clin Pathol 2006;126:564–71.

39. Leggett BA, Devereaux B, Biden K, et al. Hyperplastic polyposis: association with colorectal cancer. Am J Surg Pathol 2001;25:177–84.

40. Huang CS, O'Brien MJ, Yang S, et al. Hyperplastic polyps, serrated adenomas and the serrated polyp neoplasia pathway. Am J Gastroenterol 2004;99: 2242–55.

41. Kudo S, Lambert R, Allen JI, et al. Nonpolyposis neoplastic lesions of the colorectal mucosa. G Ital Endod 2008;68:S1–S47.

42. Brooker JC, Saunders BP, Shah SG, et al. Total colonic dye-spray increases the detection of diminutivo adenomas during routine colonoscopy: a randomized controlled trial. Gastrointest Endosc 2002;56:333–8.

43. Hurlstone DP, Cross SS, Slater R, et al. Detecting diminutive colorectal lesions at colonoscopy: a randomized controlled trial of pan-colonic versus targeted chromoscopy. Gut 2004;53:376–80.

44. Barclay RL, Vicari JJ, Doughty AS, et al. Colonoscopic withdrawal times and adenoma detection during screening colonoscopy. N Engl J Med 2006;355: 2533–41.

45. Thibodeau SN, Bren G, Schaid D. Microsatellite instability in cancer of the proximal colon. Science 1993;363:558–61.

46. Grady WM, Carethers JM. Genomic and epigenetic instability in colorectal cancer pathogenesis. Gastroenterology 2008;135:1079–99.

47. Loughrey MB, Waring PM, Tan A, et al. Incorporation of somatic BRAF mutation testing into an algorithm for the investigation of hereditary non-polyposis colorectal cancer. Fam Cancer 2007;6:301–10.

48. Gorlin RJ, Cohen MM Jr, Condon LM, et al. Bannayan-Riley-Ruvalcaba syndrome. Am J Med Genet 1992;44:307–14.

49. March DJ, Coulon V, Lunetta KL, et al. Mutation spectrum and genotype-phenotype analyses in Cowden disease and Bannayan-Zonana syndrome, two hamartoma syndromes with germline PTEN mutation. Hum Mol Genet 1998;7:507–15.

50. Eng C, Ji H. Molecular classification of the inherited hamartoma polyposis syndromes: clearing the muddied waters. Am J Hum Genet 1998;62:1020–2.

51. Marsh DJ, Kum JB, Lunetta KL, et al. PTEN mutation spectrum and genotype-phenotype correlations in Bannayan-Riley-Ruvalcaba syndrome suggest a single entity with Cowden syndrome. Hum Mol Genet 1999;8:1461–72.

52. Zbuk KM, Eng C. Hamartomatous polyposis syndromes. Nat Clin Pract Gastroenterol Hepatol 2007;4(9):492–502.

53. Zbuk KM, Stein JL, Eng C. PTEN hamartoma tumor syndrome (PHTS). Kevin M Zbuk, Jennifer L Stein, Charis Eng In: Genereviews at gene tests: medical genetics information resource [database online], University of Washington, Seattle, 1997–2006. Avaliable at: http://www.geneclinics.org. Accessed May 2009.

54. Eng C. *PTEN*: one gene, many syndromes. Hum Mutat 2003;22(3):183–98.

55. Kato M, Mizuki A, Hayash T, et al. Cowden's disease diagnosed through mucocutaneous lesions and gastrointestinal polyposis with recurrent hemorrhagic unrevealed by initial diagnosis. Intern Med 2000;39:559–63.

56. Boardman LA. Hereditable colon cancer syndromes: recognition and preventive management. Gastroenterol Clin North Am 2002;31:1107–31.

57. Haidle JL, Howe JR, Juvenile polyposis syndrome. In: Genereviews at gene tests: medical genetics information resource [database online], University of

Washington, Seattle, 1997–2006. Available at: http://www.geneclinics.org. Accessed September 9, 2008.

58. Gardlello FM, Hamilton SR, Kern SE, et al. Colorectal neoplasia in juvenile polyposis or juvenile polyps. Arch Dis Child 2001;8:319–27.

59. Heiss KF, Schaffner D, Ricketts RR, et al. Malignant risk in juvenile polyposis coli: increasing documentation in the pediatric age group. J Pediatr Surg 1993;28: 1188–93.

60. Jarvinen H, Franssila KO. Familial juvenile polyposis coli: increased risk of colorectal cancer. Gut 1984;25:792–800.

61. Howe JR, Mitros FA, Summers RW. The risk of gastrointestinal carcinoma in familial juvenile polyposis. Ann Surg Oncol 1998;5:751–6.

62. Chow E, Macrae F. A review of juvenile polyposis syndrome. J Gastroenterol Hepatol 2005;20:1634–40.

63. Brosens LAA, van Hattem A, Hylind LM, et al. Risk of colorectal cancer in juvenile polyposis. Gut 2007;56:965–7.

64. Dunlop MG. Guidance on gastrointestinal surveillance for hereditary non-polyposis colorectal cancer, familial adenomatous polyposis, juvenile polyposis, and Peutz-Jeghers syndrome. Gut 2002;51(Suppl V):v21–7.

65. Wirtzfeld DA, Petrelli NJ, Rodriquez-Bigas MA. Hamartomatous polyposis syndromes: molecular genetics, neoplastic risk and surveillance recommendations. Ann Surg Oncol 2001;8:319–27.

66. Howe JR, Roth S, Ringold JC, et al. Mutation the SMAD4/DRC4 gene in juvenile polyposis. Science 1998;280:1086–8.

67. He XL, Zhans J, Tong WG, et al. BMP signaling inhibits intestinal stem cell self-renewal through suppression of WN+-β-catenin signaling. Nat Genet 2004;36: 1117–21.

68. Howe JR, Ringold JD, Summers RW, et al. A gene for familial juvenile polyposis maps to chromosome 18q21.1. Am J Hum Genet 1998;62:1129–36.

69. Howe JR, Ringold JC, Hughes JH, et al. Direct genetic testing for SMAD4 mutations in patients at risk for juvenile polyposis. Surgery 1999;126: 162–70.

70. Howe JR, Sayed MG, Ahmed AF, et al. The prevalence of MAOH4 and BMPRIA mutations in juvenile polyposis absence of BMPR2, and ACVR1 mutations. J Med Genet 2004;41:484–91.

71. McAllister KA, Gross KM, Johnson DW, et al. Endoglin1[a] TGF-β binding protein of endothelial cells is the gene for hereditary hemorrhagic telangiectasia type 1. Nat Genet 1994;8:345–51.

72. Gallione CJ, Ropetto GM, Legins E, et al. A combined syndrome of juvenile polyposis and hereditary hemorrhagic telangiectasia associated with mutations in MADH4 (SMAD4). Lancet 2004;363:852–9.

73. Friedl W, Uhlhaas S, Schulmannk, et al. Juvenile polyposis: massive gastric polyposis is more common in MADH4 mutation carriers than in BMPRIA mutation carriers. Hum Genet 2002;111:108–11.

74. Aretz S, Stienen D, Uhlhaas S, et al. High proportion of large genomic deletions and a genotype phenotype update in 80 unrelated families with juvenile polyposis syndrome. J Med Genet 2007;44:702–9.

75. Delnatte C, Sanlaville D, Mougenot JF, et al. Contiguous gene deletion within chromosome arm 10g is associated with juvenile polyposis of infancy, reflecting cooperation between the *BMPR1A* and *PTEN* tumor-suppressor genes. Am J Hum Genet 2006;78:1066–74.

76. Salviati L, Patricelli M, Guariso G, et al. Deletion of *PTEN* and *BMPR1A* on chromosome 10g23 is not always associated with juvenile polyposis of infancy. Am J Hum Genet 2006;79:593–6.

77. Beck SE, Jung BH, Del Rosario E, et al. BMP-induced growth suppression in colon cancer cells is mediated by p21^{WAF1} stabilization and modulated by RAS/ERK. Cell Signal 2007;19:1465–72.

78. Calva-Cerqueira D, Chinnathambi S, Pechman B, et al. The rate of germline mutations and large deletions of SMAD4 and BMPR1A in juvenile polyposis. Clin Genet 2009;75(1):79–85.

79. Van Hattem WA, Brosens LA, de Leng WW, et al. Large genomic deletions of *SMAD4, BMPR1A* and *PTEN* in juvenile polyposis. Gut 2008;57(5):623–7.

80. Peutz JLA. Very remarkable case of familial polyposis of mucous membrane of intestinal tract and nasopharynx accompanied by peculiar pigmentation of skin and mucous membrane. Nederl Maandischv Genees 1921;10:134–46.

81. Jeghers H, McKusick VA, Katz KH. Generalized intestinal polyposis and melanin spots of the oral mucosa, lips, and digits: a syndrome of diagnostic significance. N Engl J Med 1949;241:993–1005.

82. Bartholemew LG, Moore CE, Dahlin DC, et al. Intestinal polyposis associated with mucocutaneous pigmentation. Surg Gynecol Obstet 1962;115:1–11.

83. Amos CI, Keitheri-Cheteri MB, Sabripour M, et al. Genotype-phenotype correlations in Peutz-Jeghers syndrome. J Med Genet 2004;41:327–33.

84. Giardiello FM, Trimbath JD. Peutz-Jeghers syndrome and management recommendations. Clin Gastroenterol Hepatol 2006;4:408–15.

85. McGarrity TJ, Amos C. Peutz-Jeghers syndrome: clinicopathology and molecular alterations. Cell Mol Life Sci 2006;63:2135–44.

86. Schulmann K, Hollerbach S, Krausk, et al. Feasibilitized diagnostic utility of video capsule endoscopy for the detection of small bowel polyposis in patients with hereditary polyposis syndrome. Am J Gastroenterol 2005;100:27–37.

87. Burke CA, Santisi J, Church J, et al. The utility of capsule endoscopy small bowel surveillance in patients with polyposis. Am J Gastroenterol 2005;100:1498–502.

88. May A, Nachbar I, Ell C. Double-balloon enteroscopy (push and pull enteroscopy) of the small bowel: feasibility and diagnostic and therapeutic yield in patients with suspected small bowel disease. Gastrointest Endosc 2005;62:62–70.

89. Ohmiya N, Tajuchi A, Chiraik, et al. Endoscopic resection of Peutz-Jeghers polyps throughout the small intestine at double-balloon enteroscopy without laparotomy. Gastrointest Endosc 2005;611:140–7.

90. Oncel M, Remzi FH, Church JM, et al. Benefits of clean sweep in Peutz-Jeghers patients. Colorectal Dis 2004;6:332–5.

91. Utsunomiya J, Gocho Miyanaga T, et al. Peutz-Jeghers syndrome: its natural course and management. Johns Hopkins Med J 1975;136(2):71–82.

92. Giardiello FM, Welsh SB, Hamilton SR, et al. Increased risk of cancer in the Peutz-Jeghers syndrome. N Engl J Med 1987;316:1511–4.

93. Spigelman AD, Arese P, Phillips RKS. Polyposis: the Peutz-Jeghers syndrome. Br J Surg 1995;82:1311–4.

94. Westerman AM, Entius MM, de Baar E, et al. Peutz-Jeghers syndrome: 78-year follow-up of the original family. Lancet 1999;353:1211–5.

95. Giardiello FM, Brensinger JD, Tersmette AC, et al. Very high risk of cancer in familial Peutz-Jeghers syndrome. Gastroenterology 2000;119:1447–53.

96. Brenster D, Raper S. synchronous colon and pancreatic cancers in a patient with Peutz-Jeghers syndrome: report of a case and review of the literature. Surgery 2004;135:352–4.

97. Hinds R, Philip C, Hyer W, et al. Complications of childhood Peutz-Jeghers syndrome: implications for pediatric screening. J Pediatr Gastroenterol Nutr 2004;39:219–20.
98. McGarrity TJ, Kulen HE, Zaino RJ. Peutz-Jeghers syndrome. Am J Gastroenterol 2000;95:596–604.
99. Lim W, Oschwang S, Keller JJ, et al. Relative frequency and morphology of cancers in STK11 mutation carriers. Gastroenterology 2004;126:1788–94.
100. Spigelman AD, Murday V, Phillips RKS. Cancer and the Peutz-Jeghers syndrome. Gut 1989;30:1588–90.
101. Foley TR, McGarrity T, Abt AB. Peutz-Jeghers syndrome: a clinicopathologic survey of the Harrisburg family with a 49-year follow-up. Gastroenterology 1988;95:1535–40.
102. Nakayama H, Fujii M, Kimura A, et al. A solitary Peutz-Jeghers-type hamartomatous polyp of the rectum: report of a case and review of the literature. Jpn J Clin Oncol 1996;26:273–6.
103. Ichyoshi Y, Yao T, Nagasaki S, et al. Solitary Peutz-Jeghers type polyp of the duodenum containing a focus of adenocarcinoma. Ital J Gastroenterol 1996; 28(2):95–7.
104. Boardman LA, Thibodeau SN, Schaid DJ, et al. Increased risk for cancer in patients with the Peutz-Jeghers syndrome. Ann Intern Med 1998;128(11):896–9.
105. Jenne DE, Reimann H, Nezu J, et al. Peutz-Jeghers syndrome is caused by mutations in a novel serine threonine kinase. Nat Genet 1998;18:38–44.
106. Hemminki A, Tomlinson I, Markie D, et al. Localization of a susceptibility locus for Peutz-Jeghers syndrome to 19p using comparative genomic hydridization and targeted linkage analysis. Nat Genet 1997;15:87–90, 94.
107. Miyoshi H, Nakau M, Ishikawa T-O, et al. Gastrointestinal hamartomatous polyposis in LKB1 heterozygous knockout mice. Cancer Res 2002;62:2261–6.

Genome-Wide Association Studies and Colorectal Cancer

Loïc Le Marchand, MD, PhD

KEYWORDS

- Colorectal cancer • Genetics • GWAS • Epidemiology
- Genetic predisposition

Colorectal cancer (CRC) is known to aggregate in families, with the disease being two- to three-times more common among the first-degree relatives of patients than in those of population controls. The contribution of inherited factors (mainly genetic) to the cause of the disease has been estimated in twin studies to be 35%.[1] However, for the most part, the underlying susceptibility genes for CRC remain unknown. In recent decades, linkage studies used collections of multicase families to identify a number of rare mutations in highly penetrant genes that cause well characterized Mendelian syndromes (eg, hereditary nonpolyposis colorectal cancer, familial adenomatous polyposis, juvenile polyposis, and Peutz-Jeghers syndrome).[2] However, these mutations explain 2% to 6% of CRCs, and only a small fraction of the familial risk. Thus, it is likely that additional susceptibility genes exist for CRC.

In recent years, linkage studies have failed to discover additional high-penetrance genes, suggesting that multiple low-penetrance alleles may explain the remaining genetic risk for CRC. Indeed, association studies, in which the frequencies of genetic variants are directly compared between large series of patients and unrelated controls, are now thought to be more appropriate than linkage studies for the identification of susceptibility loci for complex diseases, including CRC.[3]

HUMAN GENETIC VARIATION AND THE STUDY OF COMPLEX DISEASES

It is estimated that there are 10 million single-nucleotide polymorphisms (SNPs) in the human genome, half with a minor allele frequency (MAF) over 10%.[4] These genetic variants and other types of polymorphisms (insertion-deletion, copy number variations) are expected to explain approximately 90% of human heterozygosity, including susceptibility to disease.[4] Variants that were deleterious during evolution (such as mutations that cause early-onset diseases) are typically rare, owing to natural

This work was supported by grants 1R01CA126895 and 1U01HG004802 from the National Institutes of Health.

Epidemiology Program, Cancer Research Center of Hawaii, University of Hawaii, 1236 Lauhala Street, Suite 407, Honolulu, HI 96813, USA

E-mail address: loic@crch.hawaii.edu

Surg Oncol Clin N Am 18 (2009) 663–668
doi:10.1016/j.soc.2009.07.004

selection. Conversely, disease variants that act after reproduction, or that are pleio-tropic in effect, may have been neutral or subject to balancing selection (eg, sickle cell anemia and malaria). In such cases, most of the genetic variation underlying disease risk may be common.

Detailed studies of the variation in the human genome across individuals found size-able regions, or linkage disequilibrium (LD) blocks, over which little evidence for past recombination was observed, and within which more than 90% of all chromosomes matched to only one of a few common haplotypes.[5] These studies showed that nearly all of the common diversity at a given locus could be captured by genotyping a small subset of common markers.

Over the past 7 years, international efforts have resulted in a public reference human genome diversity database, a Haplotype Map of the Human Genome, which has iden-tified and validated over 3 million SNPs.[6] These resources, and the development of high-throughput microarray platforms for the simultaneous genotyping of hundreds of thousands of SNPs, now allow the testing of a high proportion of all common SNPs (with frequency $\geq 5\%$) for association with disease in studies called genome-wide association studies (GWAS). These studies allow the scanning of the entire genome for association with disease without prior knowledge of biologic function and, thus, have the potential to reveal unsuspected regions and novel biologic mech-anisms. However, theses studies require large sample sizes to account for the inflated Type-I error resulting from the very high number of case–control comparisons and to detect effect sizes that are expected to be small.

PUBLISHED GWAS OF CRC

Over the last 2 years, results from GWAS have been published for CRC. These studies have all been case-controls studies conducted in populations of European ancestry and used multistage designs.[7–13] **Table 1** summarizes the published findings from these studies as of January 2009. The risks conferred by each risk allele have uniformly been low, with odds ratios in the range of 1.1 to 1.3 per allele.[7–13]

The first susceptibility locus for CRC identified in these studies was 8q24. This genomic region first emerged for prostate cancer, through a linkage study followed up by an association study and, independently through an admixture scan in African Americans.[14,15] At least three susceptibility loci were identified for prostate cancer in 8q24.[16] One of these loci (128.1–128.7 Mb) was found to be associated with CRC in two GWAS[7,8] and, independently, in a case-control study nested in the Multiethnic Cohort study.[17] In this region, subsequently also associated with ovarian cancer, there are no known genes or annotated coding transcripts, with the exception of a pseudo-gene (*POU5F1P1*). However, approximately 300 kb telomeric to this region is the c-*MYC* (*MYC*) oncogene. Replication, sequencing, and fine-mapping studies of this locus have identified rs6983267 as the most promising variant for functional assess-ment.[18] This SNP lies in a sequence which is highly conserved across vertebrates and is predicted to have regulatory function.[18] Although *MYC* is often amplified in colon and prostate cancers, rs6983267 has not been found to modify the expression of this gene in colon tumors and lymphoblastoid cell lines. Thus, the mechanism underlying the association of this SNP to CRC and several other common cancers remains unknown. However, its relative proximity to *MYC* makes it plausible that it may disrupt one of its putative distant enhancers, the effect of which, however, may not be observable in tumors.

A locus at 9p24, also a region with no obvious candidate gene, was also found asso-ciated with CRC in the original Canadian GWAS[7] and was replicated in the Colorectal

Table 1
Characteristics of GWAS published as of January 2009 and the colorectal cancer susceptibility loci identified

Study Reference	Genotyping Platform (Nb. of SNPs)	Sample Size for Stage I	Sample Size for Subsequent Stages	Population	SNP ID (Minor Allele Frequency In Europeans)	Gene or Region	OR Per Allele	P-value Over All Sample Sets
Zanke et al[7]	Illumina and Affymetrix (99,632)	1,257 cases/1,336 controls[a]	4,024 cases/4,042 controls	First stage: Canada; Other stages: Canada, US, Scotland	rs10505477 (0.50); rs719725	8q24; 9p24	1.18; 1.14	1.41×10^{-8}; 1.32×10^{-5}
Tomlinson et al[8]	Illumina (547,647)	930 cases/960 controls[b]	7,334 cases/5,246 controls	First stage: UK; Second stage: UK	rs6983267 (0.49)	8q24	1.21	1.27×10^{-14}
Broderick et al[9]	Affymetrix (550,163)	940 cases/965 controls[b]	7,473 cases/5,984 controls	First stage: UK; Second stage: UK	rs4939827 (0.52)	18q21 SMAD7	1.18	1.0×10^{-12}
Jaeger et al[10]	Illumina (547,647)	730 cases/960 controls[b]	4,500 cases/3,860 controls	First stage: UK; Second stage: UK	rs4779584 (0.19)	15q13 CRAC1	1.26	4.4×10^{-14}
Tomlinson et al[11]	Illumina (550,163)	940 cases/965 controls[b]	17,891 cases/17,575 controls	First stage: UK; Second stage: UK, EU	rs10795668 (0.33); rs16892766 (0.07)	10p14; 8q23.3 EIF3H	0.89; 1.25	2.5×10^{-13}; 3.3×10^{-18}
Tenesa et al[12]	Illumina (541,628)	981 cases/1,002 controls[c]	16,476 cases/15,351 controls	First stage: Scotland; Second stage and replication: Canada, UK, Israel, Japan, EU	rs4939827 (0.52); rs7014346 (0.37); rs3802842 (0.29)	18q21 SMAD7; 8q24; 11q23	1.20; 1.19; 1.11	7.8×10^{-28}; 8.6×10^{-26}; 5.8×10^{-10}
Houlston et al[13]	Multiple (38,710)	6,780 cases, 6,843 controls	13,406 cases, 14,012 controls	Fist stage: UK; Replication: EU, Canada	rs4444235 (0.46); rs9929218 (0.29); rs10411210 (0.10); rs961253 (0.36)	14q22.2 BMP4; 16q22.1 CDH1; 19q13.1 RHPN2; 20p12.3	1.11; 1.20; 0.87; 1.12	8.1×10^{-10}; 1.2×10^{-8}; 4.6×10^{-9}; 2.0×10^{-10}

a Population-based controls recruited using random-digit dialing and other population-based assessment lists; matched to cases on age and sex.
b Controls were spouses or partners of European ancestry (UK resident) unaffected by cancer and without a family history of CRC.
c Controls were cancer-free and identified from the general population and matched to cases by age, sex and area of residence.

Cancer Family Registry.[19] However, since this association was not observed in some of the ARCTIC replication populations, this association may not exist in all populations.

A number of the subsequently reported loci fall within or close to a gene (18q21: *SMAD7*; 15q13.3: *CRAC1*, 8q23.3: *EIF3H*; 14q22.2: *BMP4*; 16q22.1: *CDH1*; and 19q13.1: *RHPN2*). SMAD7 is known to act as an intracellular antagonist of transforming growth factor beta signaling and perturbation of its expression had been shown to affect CRC progression.[9] EIF3H regulates cell growth and viability.[11] CRAC1 had already been linked to hereditary mixed polyposis syndrome and CRC in Ashkenazi Jews.[10] However, the other associated loci (10p14, 11q23.1, 18q23, 20p12.3), similarly to 8q24 and 9p24, lay in intergenic regions with no known biologic relevance. Thus, a large amount of work is needed to understand the biologic mechanisms underlying these associations

RESEARCH NEEDS

However, before functional studies can be initiated, resequencing and fine-mapping efforts are needed to identity the best candidate causal variants at these newly identified 11 loci. Moreover, very little information is also available on the generalization of these associations to ethic-racial groups other than whites. The only exception is rs6983267 at 8q24, which has been shown to be consistently associated with CRC among the five ethnic-racial populations in the Multiethnic Cohort (Japanese Americans, Native Hawaiians, African Americans, Whites and Latinos)[17] and to be the best candidate variants in the region.[18] Tenesa and colleagues[12] have also suggested that rs3802842 at 11q23 may not be associated with CRC in Japanese. Fine-mapping studies in populations with different linkage disequilibrium (LD) structures are potentially very useful to identify the true causal variant at a particular locus, and novel ethnic-racial–specific risk alleles.

Only limited data are available on the epidemiologic characteristics of these associations. Rs3802842 at 11q23 and rs4939827 (*SMAD7*) have been reported to be more strongly associated with rectal cancer than colon cancer.[12] No differences in risk have been reported by tumor molecular subtypes for the 11 published variants, with the exception of rs4444235 (*BMP4*) for which the association was found to be significantly stronger for mismatch repair (MMR)- proficient tumors than for MMR-deficient tumors.[13] The largest analysis conducted to date, a pooled analysis of the two United Kingdom studies, have suggested that each of the risk alleles identified so far have independent effects and that, as a group, they only explain a small proportion of cases in the population.[13] However, even in this pooled analysis, power to detect associations with SNPs having a MAF less than 0.3 was limited. This suggests that additional, somewhat less common, susceptibility variants exist and points to the need for a pooled analysis with the ongoing North American GWAS studies and the need to conduct additional GWAS.

The potential modifying effects of the newly identified susceptibility variants also need to be investigated. It is very clear from migrant and temporal trend studies that the etiology of CRC has a very strong environmental component.[20] Thus, large cohort studies, in which lifestyle risk factors for CRC were assessed before diagnosis, are being used to investigate gene-environment (GxE) interactions with the risk alleles identified in GWAS. Pooled analyses of published and existing GWAS may also provide adequate power to detect novel modifying genes in investigations of GxE interactions in the primary data.[21] Finally, populations that are especially susceptible to the effect of a Western lifestyle on CRC risk, such as the Japanese, may provide a particularly suitable population for identifying GxE interactions.[20,22]

SUMMARY

GWAS provide an efficient new approach to identify common, low-penetrance susceptibility loci without prior knowledge of biologic function. Results from GWAS conducted in populations of European ancestry living in the United Kingdom and Canada have been published for CRC. These studies have identified 11 well-replicated disease loci, which, for the majority, were not previously suspected to be related to CRC. Post-GWAS studies are being initiated to: (1) characterize the epidemiology of these associations across populations, tumor molecular sub-types, and clinically relevant variables; (2) explore GxE interactions to detect modifying effects that may explain a greater proportion of the population risk; and (3) identify the best candidate causal variants for subsequent functional studies aimed at elucidating the underlying biologic mechanisms. The proportions of the familial and population risks explained by the published loci are small and they are not currently useful for risk prediction. However, the power of the published studies was low, indicating that a number of other loci may be found in additional ongoing GWAS, especially as the result of pooled analyses of all the combined primary data. Thus, there is potential for the risk prediction ability of susceptibility markers identified in GWAS to improve as more variants are found. This may, in turn, have important implications for targeting high-risk individuals for colonoscopy screening.

REFERENCES

1. Lichtenstein P, Holm NV, Verkasalo PK, et al. Environmental and heritable factors in the causation of cancer—analyses of cohorts of twins from Sweden, Denmark and Finland. N Engl J Med 2000;343:78–85.
2. Burt RW, DiSario JA, Cannon-Albright L. Genetics of colon cancer: impact of inheritance on colon cancer risk. Annu Rev Med 1995;46:371–9.
3. Risch NJ. Searching for genetic determinants in the new millennium. Nature 2000; 405(6788):847–56.
4. Kruglyak L, Nickerson DA. Variation is the spice of life. Nat Genet 2001;27(3): 234–6.
5. Gabriel SB, Schaffner SF, Nguyen H, et al. The structure of haplotype blocks in the human genome. Science 2002;296(5576):2225–9.
6. International HapMap Consortium, Frazer KA, Ballinger DG, Cox DR, et al. A second generation human haplotype map of over 3.1 million SNPs. Nature 2007;449(7164):851–61.
7. Zanke BW, Greenwood CM, Rangrej J, et al. Genome-wide association scan identifies a colorectal cancer susceptibility locus on chromosome 8q24. Nat Genet 2007;39(8):989–94.
8. Tomlinson I, Webb E, Carvajal-Carmona L, et al. A genome-wide association scan of tag SNPs identifies a susceptibility variant for colorectal cancer at 8q24.21. Nat Genet 2007;39(8):984–8.
9. Broderick P, Carvajal-Carmona L, Pittman AM, et al. A genome-wide association study shows that common alleles of SMAD7 influence colorectal cancer risk. Nat Genet 2007;39(11):1315–7.
10. Jaeger E, Webb E, Howarth K, et al. Common genetic variants at the CRAC1 (HMPS) locus on chromosome 15q13.3 influence colorectal cancer risk. Nat Genet 2008;40(1):26–8.
11. Tomlinson IP, Webb E, Carvajal-Carmona L, et al. A genome-wide association study identifies colorectal cancer susceptibility loci on chromosomes 10p14 and 8q23.3. Nat Genet 2008;40(5):623–30.

12. Tenesa A, Farrington SM, Prendergast JG, et al. Genome-wide association scan identifies a colorectal cancer susceptibility locus on 11q23 and replicates risk loci at 8q24 and 18q21. Nat Genet 2008;40(5):631–7.
13. Houlston RS, Webb E, Broderick P, et al. Meta-analysis of genome-wide association data identifies four new susceptibility loci for colorectal cancer. Nat Genet 2008;40(12):1426–35.
14. Amundadottir LT, Sulem P, Gudmundsson J, et al. A common variant associated with prostate cancer in European and African populations. Nat Genet 2006;38(6): 652–8.
15. Freedman ML, Haiman CA, Patterson N, et al. Admixture mapping identifies 8q24 as a prostate cancer risk locus in African-American men. Proc Natl Acad Sci U S A 2006;103(38):14068–73.
16. Haiman C, Patterson N, Freedman ML, et al. Three regions within 8q24 independently modulate risk for prostate cancer. Nat Genet 2007;39:638–44.
17. Haiman CA, Le Marchand L, Yamamato J, et al. A common genetic risk factor for colorectal and prostate cancer. Nat Genet 2007;39(8):954–6.
18. Yeager M, Xiao N, Hayes RB, et al. Comprehensive resequence analysis of a 136 kb region of human chromosome 8q24 associated with prostate and colon cancers. Hum Genet 2008;124(2):161–70.
19. Poynter JN, Figueiredo JC, Conti DV, et al. Variants on 9p24 and 8q24 are associated with risk of colorectal cancer: results from the Colon Cancer Family Registry. Cancer Res 2007;67(23):11128–32.
20. Le Marchand L, Wilkens LR. Design considerations for genomic association studies: importance of gene-environment interactions. Cancer Epidemiol Biomarkers Prev 2008;17(2):263–7.
21. Evans DN, Marchini J, Morris AP, et al. Two-stage two-locus models in genome-wide association. PLoS Genet 2006;2:1424–32.
22. Le Marchand L. Combined influence of genetic and dietary factors on colorectal cancer incidence in Japanese Americans. J Natl Cancer Inst Monogr 1999;26: 101–5.

Genetic Counseling for Hereditary Colorectal Cancer: Ethical, Legal, and Psychosocial Issues

Melyssa Aronson, MS, CCGC, CGC

KEYWORDS

• Genetic counseling • Ethical • Legal • Psychosocial
• Duty-to-warn • Testing minors

The impression that genetic testing for an inherited colorectal cancer (CRC) syndrome involves a simple blood test masks the complex issues that surround this type of testing. This article explores the ethical, legal, and psychosocial implications of genetic testing and the role of genetic counseling through the genetic testing process.

WHAT IS A GENETIC COUNSELOR?

Genetic counseling is defined as "the process of helping people understand and adapt to the medical, psychological and familial implications of genetic conditions to disease."[1] Genetic counselors are health professionals with a specialized degree in genetics and counseling. They work with a multidisciplinary team to counsel people who have personal or family histories suspicious of an inherited syndrome. Patients are often referred through family physicians, specialists, or by self-referral. Locating a genetic counselor by geographic area can be achieved by searching the Web sites of the National Society of Genetic Counselors (NSGC) (http://www.nsgc.org); the Canadian Association for Genetic Counsellors (http://www.cagc-accg.ca); or the Collaborative Group of the Americas on Inherited Colorectal Cancer (http://www.cgaicc.com). A more complete list of available Web sites has been outlined in a genetic counseling review article by Dr. Lynch.[2]

THE GENETIC COUNSELING PROCESS

The proband meets with a genetic counselor for risk assessment and to gather information to make an informed decision about genetic testing. The NSGC

Department of Surgery, Mount Sinai Hospital, 60 Murray Street, Box 24, Toronto, Ontario M5T 3L9, Canada
E-mail address: maronson@mtsinai.on.ca (M. Aronson).

Surg Oncol Clin N Am 18 (2009) 669–685
doi:10.1016/j.soc.2009.07.001
1055-3207/09/$ – see front matter © 2009 Elsevier Inc. All rights reserved.

surgonc.theclinics.com

outlines 12 elements that should be discussed as part of the informed consent process:[3]

1. Purpose of the test and who to test
2. General information about the genes
3. Possible test results (positive, uninformative, informative negative, unclassified variant of unknown significance)
4. Likelihood of positive result
5. Technical aspects and accuracy of the test
6. Economic considerations
7. Risks of genetic discrimination
8. Psychosocial aspects
9. Confidentiality issues
10. Use of test results: medical surveillance and preventative measures
11. Alternatives to genetic testing
12. Storage and potential reuse of genetic material

An accepted genetic counseling protocol consists of a pretest session and a result session with further follow-up as needed.[4,5] Obtaining family history information and medical records before the pretest session aids in the initial assessment and the outline of the session. Decision aids have also been reported to facilitate the decision-making process for patients undergoing testing for Lynch syndrome.[6]

The pretest counseling session is outlined in great detail in this article, along with the ethical, legal, and psychosocial implications of genetic testing. The focus is on the pretest session because much of the information gathered during this session guides discussions in the posttest session. The posttest session often involves disclosing and interpreting results, reviewing preventative surveillance and surgical recommendations, discussing the impact results may have on kin and the importance of disclosure to family members, exploring the psychosocial impact of the result, and referring to other specialists and support groups as required. After results are disclosed, the genetic counselor follows-up with the proband as needed and may encourage the proband to contact the clinic if changes in the family occur that may affect the risk assessment, or to update themselves on new genetic data that continue to emerge.

PRETEST GENETIC COUNSELING SESSION

The pretest session is outlined in three sections: (1) risk assessment; (2) educational component; and (3) issues surrounding the ethical, legal, and psychosocial implications of genetic testing. The process of contracting at the beginning of the session allows both genetic counselor and proband to express their intentions for the session and outline a plan that meets both expectations. Suggestions for information to be gathered are outlined in each section with the understanding that these are not meant to be exhaustive and each genetic counseling session must be tailored to meet the needs of the proband and the policies of the clinic.

Risk Assessment

Family history
Although patients with classical familial adenomatous polyposis (FAP) present clinically with a recognizable phenotype, assessing most families for inherited CRC syndromes is not as obvious. To assess the family properly, a three- to four-generation pedigree should be constructed. Ideally, the family history can be gathered from a completed questionnaire sent to the proband in advance of the pretest session.

As with all genetic conditions, questions regarding ethnicity, consanguinity, and other genetic conditions and testing in the family should be asked.

Specific information should be gathered on the cancer diagnoses in the family, including the type of cancer, age of diagnoses, and current age or age of death. Enquiring about the year of diagnosis and hospital of surgery may indicate whether tumor tissue, often needed for microsatellite instability (MSI) and immunohistochemistry testing, is still available. Enquires should also be made about current and past surveillance and surgeries (e.g. hysterectomy); polyp history; and coexisting conditions that predispose to CRC, such as inflammatory bowel disease. Because probands may not associate benign findings with an inherited CRC syndrome, they should be asked directly about associated features for the syndrome being investigated, such as skin lesions associated with Lynch syndrome or freckling associated with Peutz-Jeghers syndrome. As part of the assessment, other risk factors, such as smoking, alcohol consumption, and occupation risks, should be queried.

The cancer and noncancer information reported by the proband may be more accurate among their first-degree relatives than in more distant kin. Inaccuracies have also been reported when probands give information about relatives in older generations; synchronous tumors; and certain site-specific cancers, such as stomach, ovarian, and urinary tract cancers.[7,8] CRC diagnoses have also been reported inaccurately, even among first-degree relatives.[9,10] Glanz and colleagues[10] reported confirming CRC in parents and siblings in 25% of families where no cancer was reported in the proband's first-degree relatives. Predictors of inaccurate reporting included relatives with low knowledge of CRC and males in the family. The best predictor for accuracy was the stage of CRC at diagnosis. Patients with higher knowledge of the disease, with increased perceived risk and cancer worry, and with better communication in the family tended to report CRC more accurately.

Family history should be interpreted with caution and every effort should be made to obtain pathology confirmation. If medical records are unavailable, the genetic counselor should review the limitations of the assessment in the absence of confirmation of cancer and reiterate that the risk may change if new information is gathered.

Confirmation of medical records

Pathology reports should be obtained to confirm malignant and benign diagnoses whenever possible. Specifics about the age of diagnosis, cancer site and stage, type of surgery, presence of metachronous and synchronous tumors, presence and histology of polyps, and features associated with MSI status, (eg, tumor-infiltrating lymphocytes, mucinous, signet cell ring, Crohn's-like lymphocytic reaction) can be extracted from the pathology report and medical records.

To obtain medical records, clinics may have the affected individual or their next-of-kin sign an authorization to release records from the health care facility where surgery or endoscopy was performed. Authorization forms may also be needed to acquire tumor tissue for preliminary genetic testing. Because MSI and immunohistochemistry have been likened to other medical screening tests that do not require written authorization, Gaff and colleagues[11] examined the protocols for consent to obtain tissue samples in the United Kingdom. They found that most clinics obtained authorization from affected individuals to test their tumor samples, although relatives of the consultant may not have been seen in-person for consent. Less than half of the clinics obtained consent from next-of-kin to test a sample from a deceased individual, although legislation was not in place at the time to regulate obtaining consent to test stored tissue. The authors suggested that MSI and immunohistochemistry testing should constitute its own niche between a screening and diagnostic test and discussions are needed regarding the acceptable practices for genetic counseling and consent.

The family history and medical records should be carefully evaluated. Risk assessment models and protocols for genetic testing of suspected inherited CRC syndromes are discussed elsewhere in this issue.

Educational Component

As part of the educational component of the session, the counselor should review the genetics of CRC and outline the conditions being investigated in the family. A review of the genetic and clinical aspects of that condition should include information on the inheritance, cancer penetrance, and other clinical features of the disease; cancer surveillance; and preventative strategies. The use of chemoprevention and lifestyle modifications should be discussed if appropriate. Based on the risk assessment, the proband should be informed of the likelihood of having the condition being investigated. A full review of the genetic testing process should be described, including the pros and cons and alternatives to undergoing testing.

The pretest session is also an appropriate time to discuss possible outcomes of a genetic test and the implications for the family. Initiating discussions about disseminating results to at-risk family members during this session has been observed to lead to the best outcome in actual disclosure to relatives.[12] This may be caused by the fact that probands can begin to prepare their relatives for the possibility of receiving genetic test results and allow their kin to decline being informed if that is their desire. It also allows probands to formulate a plan for disseminating information to their family members, which can be supported with written material provided by the genetic clinic.

Legal, Ethical, and Psychosocial Issues

This section explores the different issues that can impact a proband's risk perceptions, motivations and barriers to undergo testing, coping and adjustment to results, disseminating information to relatives, and others issues that families undergoing genetic testing for inherited CRC conditions may contemplate.

Impact of cancer in the family

As part of the pedigree review, genetic counselors should encourage probands to share their experiences with cancer by relaying their diagnosis story and by describing the cancer burden they have felt in the family. This experiential knowledge has been shown to impact a person's perception of risk, cancer worry, and the ability to understand information being relayed in the counseling session.[13–15] If, for example, screening colonoscopy failed to detect a malignancy in the family, this may impact the proband's trust in surveillance if one day faced with the decision to continue surveillance or consider prophylactic surgery.

Probands have also been found to have personal theories of inheritance based on observations in their family. They may be convinced that an autosomal genetic condition is gender-linked if the cancer runs predominantly with one gender in the family. There are also theories of codominant inheritance linked to a certain blood type or physical feature that, by happenstance, is common among all carriers of the disease.[16]

By gaining an understanding of how cancer has impacted the proband, the genetic counselor can better prepare how to relay information and facilitate discussion within the family.

Motivations and deterrents for genetic testing

The decision to undergo testing has often been reached before the pretest genetic counseling session.[4,6,17] Studies have shown that patients are interested in genetic testing for cancer genetic syndromes,[17,18] but the overall uptake for Lynch syndrome testing has been found to be lower than anticipated based on expressed interest.[19,20]

Strong motivators for probands to undergo genetic testing include the desire to define the risk to their children and to determine appropriate cancer-reducing strategies for themselves.[17,19,21] One of the strongest motivators is the relief from uncertainty, especially by learning that an at-risk relative is not a carrier.[19,22] To a lesser extent, probands may also wish to have testing to make decisions regarding reproductive and family planning.[19]

Probands who undergo genetic testing tend to have a higher risk perception of developing cancer or of inheriting the genetic predisposition, and believe they are better able to cope with the results and comply with surveillance recommendations.[17,23] There have been inconsistencies observed on the impact that gender and age has on the decision to pursue genetic testing.[17,19,23,24]

Because higher risk perception is a motivator for testing, and probands from families meeting Amsterdam criteria do feel a higher risk of carrying a mutation compared with those not fulfilling the criteria,[21] the question arises whether a strong family history is predictive of who undergoes genetic testing. Studies have shown conflicting results regarding the correlation between family history and uptake of genetic testing.[13,17,18,19,20,23] In families considered high-risk or with confirmed Lynch syndrome, some studies have reported less than half the probands proceed with genetic testing.[19,20,23] This may be suggestive of an avoidance reaction related to the anxiety and distress associated with a high-risk perception of having a genetic mutation.

Deterrents to genetic testing include concerns about the loss of health insurance, impact on the family, and the psychologic impact of a positive result.[17,19,22] Probands who are less likely to partake in genetic testing include those with less formal education; depression identified during pretest session; avoiders of medical screening (e.g. colonoscopy); and those who feel unable to deal with results.[17,20,23]

Genetic counselors should have an understanding of the motivations and barriers to genetic testing and be prepared to outline the potential benefits and limitations for their consultant as an essential part of the informed consent process.

Genetic discrimination

Hadley and colleagues[17] reported that almost 40% of individuals contemplating genetic testing for Lynch syndrome stated that the fear of genetic discrimination was the primary deterrent to undergoing genetic testing. This may explain why only 51% of first-degree relatives in families with known mutations decided to pursue predictive testing. A low percentage of uptake (43%) was seen in two additional American studies of first-degree relatives in high-risk and mutation-positive families,[20,23] which is in sharp contrast to observations in a Finnish study that reported a 75% rate of uptake among relatives.[22] It was speculated by the Finnish authors that the discrepancy may be caused by the difference in health care systems, because individuals in Finland have access to universal health care and are less concerned over insurance discrimination compared with individuals in the United States.

Since the time of those studies, a law known as the Genetic Information Nondiscrimination Act was passed in the United States and it is expected to go into effect in 2009. The law prohibits insurers from requiring that customers undergo genetic testing before acquiring insurance, nor can they use prior knowledge of a genetic test result to deny or set high premiums. It also prohibits employers from asking employees about their genetic status or using such information in their hiring or other employment decisions. Some limitations of the Genetic Information Nondiscrimination Act are that the insurance protection does not apply to patients already manifesting symptoms related to the cancer syndrome, and the law does not apply to employers with less than 15 employees or to members of the United States Military.[25]

Despite the concern over genetic discrimination, a study of patients with FAP reported that only 16% of them experienced discrimination, mostly related to employment because of increase needs to use the washroom, absence from work for surveillance, and physical limitations.[26] The actual impact of genetic discrimination on individuals undergoing genetic testing for susceptibility syndromes is not clear and may need to be re-evaluated once the Genetic Information Nondiscrimination Act has taken effect. The fear of genetic discrimination may be a barrier for some individuals considering genetic testing and should be raised by the genetic counselor as a potential limitation to genetic testing.

Psychologic impact of genetic testing

There have been several studies investigating the psychologic impact of genetic testing for Lynch syndrome. Although an increase in intrusive thoughts and fears about cancer, depression, and anxiety have been measured immediately following a positive results, these levels have returned to baseline at the 1-year follow-up.[20,27–30]

Esplen and colleagues[21] identified factors associated with postcounseling distress including perceived lower satisfaction with social support, an escape-avoidant coping style, and anticipation of being depressed if a mutation was identified. The authors observed that individuals who anticipate they have a mutation are better able to cope with positive results because they are already engaged in active coping strategies. A difference was noted in distress levels between carriers who have had a previous diagnosis of cancer compared with nonaffected carriers, with the latter being more vulnerable to psychologic distress immediately following disclosure of a positive result. This distress was attributed to the fact that an unaffected relative not only has to adjust to a potentially unanticipated result, but also to an increased risk of developing cancer.[31]

In the event of a positive result, probands report having increased concern for children and guilt for passing on a mutation. They also report plans to make healthier lifestyle choices.[13,21] There may also be an impact on familial relationships, family planning, and a different outlook on life than there was before results were disclosed.[13]

For probands who are found to be informative negative (i.e. confirmed not to carry the familial mutation) there is a sense of relief that results in decrease of intrusive and avoidant thoughts of CRC and depression.[29] Probands undergoing genetic testing for Lynch syndrome can be reassured that there have been no adverse psychologic outcomes reported among patients who tested positive for Lynch syndrome.[30]

In contrast, individuals undergoing genetic testing for FAP may have adverse outcomes after genetic testing. Douma and colleagues[32] reported in a recent review article that clinical anxiety or depression has been reported in individuals after undergoing genetic testing for FAP. Similar to Lynch syndrome, however, there is an interest in genetic testing primarily to relieve uncertainty and to assess individual risk and the risk to offspring.

Young adults and adolescents who underwent genetic testing for FAP expressed feeling concern for their parent, anger, regret about knowing they have the mutation, distance from family members, guilt over negative result, and anxiety. An awareness of true friendships, relief from uncertainty, bonding with other affected family members, and feeling a sense of control were some of the benefits of undergoing testing.[33]

Patients with FAP have also reported distress in regard to body image and sexual and physical functioning, correlating strongly with patients who underwent an ileal-pouch anal anastomosis.[34,35] Patients who were single at the time of surgery were also found to be more vulnerable to psychologic distress compared with their married counterparts.[34,36]

The psychologic implications of genetic testing must be addressed during the counseling sessions and additional support may be needed for individuals who are more susceptible to anxiety and distress. The clinical manifestation of the syndrome, extent of surveillance, and surgical intervention, along with the perceived risk, coping style, and level of distress in the patient should be considered when reviewing the different inherited CRC syndromes.

Testing of minors

The American Society of Clinical Oncology's (ASCO) policy statement reports that, with parental involvement, consideration be given to testing minors for conditions associated with cancer in childhood that have evidence-based risk-reduction strategies.[37] Research has found that clinical geneticists would support this recommendation by offering genetic testing for children at risk for FAP as young as 6 years old.[38] The main justification for predictive and presymptomatic genetic testing of an unaffected minor is if there is available medical intervention or preventative measures in childhood.[39] Andrews and colleagues[26] reported that 42% of patients with FAP believed that genetic testing for children should be available "at birth" with one parent quoted as saying, "[It] should be the right of the parent to decide what age [children] can be tested, not the Hereditary Cancer Registry to dictate the rights of someone else's life." This was supported by the observations of Whitelaw and colleagues[40] who found 93.5% of parents would want their children tested for FAP at birth.

Despite the fact that medical intervention is not necessary at birth, parents' desire for relief from the uncertainty and guilt and eliminating unnecessary screening in children not at-risk is suggested as the reasons for wanting the test so early in life. The policy of most clinics is to offer predictive testing between the ages of 11 and 15, and parents generally agree that this is the most appropriate age to begin discussions of FAP with their children.[26,40]

Studies have shown that children undergoing testing for FAP do not suffer significant psychologic issues as a result of genetic testing, although they do worry more than children who tested negative. Children with siblings who have tested positive for FAP were more vulnerable to adverse outcomes.[35,41,42]

In regard to cancer syndromes that predispose to adult-onset malignancy, ASCO recommends deferring genetic testing until the minor is of an age that they can make an informed decision about the testing.[37] Borry and colleagues[39] reviewed 27 ethical and clinical guidelines and position papers concerning the presymptomatic and predictive genetic testing of minors and the consensus was to recommend that testing be deferred for adult-onset disorders until the minor was old enough to consent as a competent adolescent or adult. A survey of clinicians concurred because they were cautious regarding testing children and adolescents (age 16) for syndromes that would not have a direct-medical benefit in childhood.[38]

Prenatal screening and preimplantation genetic diagnosis

Patients with FAP have reported refraining from having biologic children because of the fear of passing on the familial mutation.[40,43] Similarly, 40% of patients with

Peutz-Jeghers syndrome reported altering their reproductive choices based on their diagnosis.[44] Prenatal screening, including amniocentesis, chorionic villous sampling (CVS), and preimplantation genetic diagnosis (PGD) can identify transmission of disease to offspring at the earliest stages of development. CVS and amniocentesis occur during pregnancy between weeks 10 and 12 and 16 and 20, respectively. Both tests can identify genetic mutations carried by the fetus and are associated with a small risk of miscarriage (approximately 1% and 0.5%, respectively). As implied, PGD occurs before pregnancy and involves analyzing an amplified polar body (if disease is maternally transmitted) or one to two cells from an eight-cell embryo retrieved through the in vitro fertilization process to identify and reimplant embryos that do not carry the familial mutation.

Offit and colleagues[45] explored some of the psychologic, social, and ethical controversies involved with PGD. Ethically, there remains controversy over the types of conditions in which PGD should be offered. There is also the issue of the outcome of embryos found to carry the genetic mutation. Concerns over misdiagnoses and potential imprinting defects associated with the process have been raised. Socially, there is the issue of cost, which makes this option unattainable for some couples and those that can afford it may face low success rates through the in vitro fertilization process. For some couples, however, the option of PGD is advantageous when faced with the possibility of pregnancy termination of an affected fetus.

PGD has been used to identify embryos carrying both MMR and *APC* gene mutations.[46,47] Controversy remains over the use of PGD for adult-onset disorders that are more commonly associated with incomplete penetrance and a higher likelihood of cancer prevention through surveillance and prophylactic surgery. Prenatal testing for early onset conditions, such as FAP, is more widely accepted, because of the impact in childhood, the complete penetrance of the disease, and the inevitable surgical intervention.

Studies have shown that most patients with or at-risk for FAP would consider the option of prenatal testing.[26,40,43] In 1996, even before prenatal testing was available, Whitelaw and colleagues[40] found 65% of patients would consider prenatal testing, and 24% would terminate a child with FAP. Kastrinos and colleagues[43] reported in a pilot study of 20 patients with FAP that 95% of them would consider prenatal testing: 90% would consider PGD and 75% would consider amniocentesis or CVS. This was higher than a study of 88 patients by Andrews and colleagues,[26] where 75% would consider prenatal testing and 61.4% would consider PGD. Twenty-one percent reported that they would elect to terminate an affected pregnancy. Individuals preferred PGD over amniocentesis or CVS because it allowed them to feel reassured from the start of the pregnancy that the fetus was unaffected, without needing to consider the option of elective termination of pregnancy.[43]

The genetic counselor can facilitate conversation for parents who are of reproductive age and considering the option of prenatal testing. Beginning these discussions during the pretest session allows probands to ponder their options and begin discussions with their partner before receiving a positive result.

Disclosure of results

Because of the inherited nature of a genetic disorder, a deleterious mutation identified in an individual has implications for all members of the family. Overall, CRC patients believe it is important to share genetic information with their family.[21,48,49] In a population-based study of CRC patients in Ontario, Canada, undergoing genetic testing for Lynch syndrome, 93% believed it was their duty to inform relatives of genetic test results. Specifically, 91.3% anticipated telling their spouse about a mutation, 88.3%

would tell their offspring, and 70% would disclose results to more distant relatives and friends.[21] Similar findings were reported from the Seattle Colorectal Cancer Family Registry where 100% of cases believed they would disclose results to their spouse, children, and siblings.[18] Both studies reported most patients and relatives also anticipated sharing results with their family physician.

The anticipated intention of open communication has been confirmed by probands once results were received.[24,50] Stoffel and colleagues[50] reported that 98% of individuals with Lynch syndrome shared results with their first-degree relatives including their children. Sixty-seven percent reported sharing results with second- or third-degree relatives, associated more so with probands who had a very strong family history of cancer. If a deleterious mutation was identified, 75% of participants reported sharing results with second- or third-degree relatives. Probands were more apt to share results if they wished to encourage at-risk family members to have testing and if they required support from family members.

Other motivators of disclosure included feelings of moral obligation, family duty, and a responsibility for the health of others, with probands expressing regret if a cancer were to occur that could have been otherwise prevented.[24,51]

Reasons given for not disclosing results to relatives included estranged relationships or little contact with kin, avoidance, fear of genetic discrimination, and concern over misinterpretation of results by kin.[13,48,50,52] The age of the proband and the relative may also impact disclosure. Probands who were young were less likely to communicate results and overall, individuals were less likely to disclose results to elderly relatives.[48,51] Another deterrent to open communication occurred if the first attempt to share information in the family was a negative experience.[51] Probands were wary of causing concern in the family and reported that bereavement and recent diagnoses or death in the family also presented barriers to disseminating information.[13,24,50]

Concern over the reaction of relatives prompts the argument that by disclosing results to unsuspecting relatives, it removes their autonomous right to decline being informed of the condition in the family. When asked about disclosure of results to family, one individual undergoing Lynch syndrome testing was quoted to say, "The one who is 'telling' has invaded the hearer's privacy."[48] Despite the concerns, studies have reported that relatives do wish to be informed about a genetic risk in the family.[18,49,53,54]

Most families believed a personal approach is the preferred method of disclosure of results to relatives.[49,51] Pentz and colleagues[49] reported that although most relatives preferred to be informed by their relatives, 20% believed it was the duty of the health care profession to disclose risk information to the family. One relative was quoted to say, "I think it comes back to the Hippocratic Oath. The first law is to do no harm. If to say nothing is to do harm, then I think you have an obligation to pass the information on." Seventy-six percent of relatives believed it was permissible for the health care provider to disclose results to family members, and very few qualified that by saying that permission should first be obtained from the proband. The relatives were cognizant of breaching confidentiality, but suggested that the provider could simply say a mutation was identified in the family without revealing the identity of the individual who underwent testing. If the identity of the proband was not revealed, then relatives believed the knowledge of the risk information outweighs the concerns about confidentiality.

Probands have agreed with the notion that health care providers could provide information to family members. In a study by Kohut and colleagues[48] over 73% of CRC probands being investigated for Lynch syndrome would allow their genetic counselor or physician to warn their family members about a genetic risk and 55.8% agreed with the statement "I would want my physician or genetic counselor to tell certain family members (whom I did not feel comfortable telling) that I had an HNPCC mutation, even without my permission."

Atkan-Collan and colleagues[55] designed a direct-approach method to contact relatives in Lynch syndrome families identified through the Finnish hereditary nonpolyposis colorectal cancer registry. They found 51% of relatives agreed to counseling and 92% were satisfied with the approach method. Of those relatives, 40% pursued testing and on first postresult colonoscopy, 11 out of 32 carriers were found to have neoplasia including four cancers and seven adenomatous polyps.

It has been shown that relatives would want to be informed of a familial disease that was probable, serious, and treatable even if it was against the proband's wishes.[53]

Physician's duty-to-warn

If a patient refuses to inform their at-risk relatives of a genetic condition in the family, the genetic counselor and treating physician must struggle between their duty to respect the autonomy and confidentiality of their patient against the ethical principles of nonmaleficence and beneficence for at-risk relatives.

Two landmark American court cases outline rulings over the physician's duty to warn relatives of a genetic predisposition in the family. The case of Pate v Threlkel (1995) involved a law suit against Dr. Threlkel who failed to warn Ms. Pate of her mother's diagnosis of hereditary medullary thyroid cancer. The Florida Supreme Court ruled that Dr. Threlkel had a duty to warn the at-risk relative; however, this duty would be fulfilled by informing the parent of the risk to their child.[56] In the case of Safer v Pack (1996), Ms. Safer filed a suit against her father's physician, the late Dr. Pack, claiming she was not warned of her father's diagnosis of FAP. In contrast to the decision in Pate v Threlkel, the New Jersey appellate court ruled the physician must take "reasonable steps" to warn at-risk family members thereby extending the physician's duty-to-warn beyond simply informing their patient of the risk to their kin. The court did not address the issue of confidentiality, nor did it provide specific recommendations as to how a physician should disseminate this information.[57]

Different organizations have created policy statements regarding duty-to-warn. ASCO believes the provider is best used by encouraging communication within the family and emphasizing to the patient the importance and benefit of sharing the genetic information with their at-risk relatives.[37] Similarly, the NSGC believes it is the patient's right to decide who has access to their results.[58]

The statement by the American Medical Association is more forceful, stating, "Physicians also should identify circumstances under which they would expect patients to notify biologic relatives of the availability of information related to risk of disease. In this regard, physicians should make themselves available to assist patients in communicating with relatives to discuss opportunities for counseling and testing, as appropriate."[59]

Although there have been no liability suits in Canada,[60,61] the Canadian Medical Association's Code of Ethics states that a physician can only disclose their patient's information with consent, unless the "maintenance of confidentiality would result in a significant risk of substantial harm to others or, in the case of incompetent patients, to the patients themselves. In such cases take all reasonable steps to inform the patients that the usual requirements for confidentiality will be breached."[62]

The American Society of Human Genetics (ASHG) takes a more directive approach than the American Medical Association and Canadian Medical Association by stating that in a situation where all attempts at communication in the family have failed, and "harm is highly likely to occur and is serious and foreseeable; where the at-risk relative(s) is identifiable; and where either the disease is preventable, treatable, or medically accepted standards indicate that early monitoring will reduce the genetic risk," then disclosure should be permissible.[63] Of interest, one study found that only 38% of medical geneticists were aware of ASHG's policy on disclosure.[52]

The policy by ASHG is in accordance with the American Privacy Act, Health Insurance Portability and Accountability Act of 1996, which prohibits clinicians from breaching patient confidentiality unless there is a "serious and imminent threat to the health or safety of a person or the public."[64] This too is in line with the Canadian's Personal Health Information Protection Act and Quality of Care Information Protection Act, which came into effect in November, 2004, and states that health care professionals must obtain consent to share health care information "except in specific circumstances where the law authorizes health care providers to collect, use or share a person's information without consent, such as reporting for public health safety."[65]

Physicians contemplating duty-to-warn struggle with the meaning of the words "serious" and "imminent threat" when referring to susceptibility conditions with incomplete penetrance. Furthermore, despite the cancer risk being greatly increased over the general population risk, surveillance recommendations can be established for individuals at high-risk, even in the absence of genetic test results, thereby reducing their actual risk of developing cancer.

Offit and colleagues[66] stated in a review paper that "clinicians need to balance the actual risk of that disease, the efficacy of potential preventive interventions, as well as emerging legal considerations and potential liabilities. Overriding patient confidentiality and genetic privacy might very well mean violation of HIPAA and certain state regulations, with attendant civil or criminal liability." The authors acknowledged the legal precedence as reviewed previously; however, they argued that the policies outlined by ASCO and the American Medical Association represent the most practical approach for physicians. Physicians were recommended to carefully document discussions regarding this issue as part of both the pretest and posttest counseling session.

Forrest and colleagues[67] reviewed 19 guidelines from six countries, mainly in Europe and Australia, regarding communication of genetic information in families. Overall, the guidelines encouraged providers to educate their consultants about the importance of disseminating information to at-risk family members. Few policies instructed the provider to identify the at-risk relatives for the proband or to provide them with supportive written material. Only three organizations addressed the option for the provider to disclose results at the request of the patient. In contrast to the nondirective approach used by most geneticists and genetic counselors, most policies encourage a directive approach in regard to discussions on family disclosure. One notable exception was from the German Society of Human Genetics stating, "Geneticists who press for the information to be relayed violate patient autonomy."

The inconsistencies in policy recommendations were also noted by Godard and colleagues[68] who reviewed 62 international guidelines. The authors divided the policies into those who would allow physician disclosure (1) with patient consent only, (2) without patient's consent, or (3) under exceptional circumstances. They highlighted several organizations and countries that did not allow for communication between physician and third parties, including France, whose law mandates strict confidentiality. The Danish Council of Ethics and ASCO were also singled out as having policies that limited the physician's involvement only to their patient. A comprehensive list of all policy statements can be found in the review article.

Although the policies are not consistent, geneticists overwhelmingly report encouraging their consultants to disclose results in a family. Despite these recommendations, most medical geneticists and genetic counselors have encountered nondisclosure in the family (60% and 46%, respectively). Sixty-nine percent of medical geneticists feel responsible to warn their patient's at-risk relative; however, only 20% to 25% of genetic counselors and geneticist seriously considered disclosing results directly to relatives and very few admitted following through with that decision.[52,69] Geneticists report patient confidentiality, the patient-physician relationship, ethical and legal concerns, institutional policies, and the hope of an eventual resolution in the family as reasons to avoid disclosure without the patient's consent.[52]

When given a scenario highlighting the issue of duty-to-warn a second-degree relative in a family with a known MMR mutation, the NSGC ethics subcommittee believed the obligation of the counselor was to inform the proband of the risk to kin and to provide supportive material and resources that can aid in disclosure.[70] Chan-Smutko and colleagues[12] also outlined a scenario featuring nondisclosure involving a woman with endometrial cancer and a known *MSH6* mutation who did not wish to share her results with her unaffected sister. This scenario was complicated by the fact that one physician was treating both siblings and was aware that mutation information was not being shared. In this scenario, the physician recommended that the unaffected sibling proceed with comprehensive testing based solely on her strong family history. A further complication was added when the insurance company denied the claim for the more expensive test in an unaffected individual. If the mutation information was known, a less expensive predictive test would have been available. Although the physician was able to resolve the problem in the family by encouraging communication between the sisters, the authors argued that in this situation the conditions set forth by the ASHG have been met; however, they contend that the term "serious" is subjective and "foreseeable" may be argued because penetrance is not 100%.

Given the complex issues at hand, the genetic counselor can be instrumental in educating the individual undergoing genetic testing about the implications results may have on family members. By initiating this conversation during the pretest session, the consultant can begin to consider the issue of disclosing results to at-risk relatives before testing. Concerns of the proband can be addressed and written material can be provided to the proband to assist in disseminating information. Genetic counselors can make themselves available to family members who contact them with questions or who wish to be referred to a genetic counselor in their area. If caregivers find themselves in a situation where all other tactics have failed, they may work toward resolution by speaking with their colleagues and ethic boards and consult their institution's policy on duty-to-warn.[52]

Direct-to-consumer testing

With the advancement of genetic technology using copy number variants and single nucleotide polymorphisms, the understanding of lower penetrance inherited CRC syndromes is expanding. Commercial laboratories are benefiting from this new technology by advertising directly to consumers, offering genetic testing through a simple cheek swab that can be mailed away and interpreted for a price.

Wasson and colleagues[71] reviewed many of the ethical issues that have been raised in response to this new wave of consumer genetic testing. There is little regulation of the direct-to-consumer testing companies (DTC) who may or may not meet stringent federal certifications. It may also be impossible for the company to verify whether the DNA being tested belongs to the person completing the paperwork. Because consumers are not directed to speak with a genetic specialist, they may not be aware of the benefits and limitations of the testing, or the implications it may have on themselves or their family. Once results are received, the consumer may have difficulty interpreting them and given that the sensitivity and specificity of the testing is not well established, the accuracy of the results may be in question. The consumers' need to have their result interpreted by their family doctor or genetic specialist may put undue stress on an already overburdened medical profession. Based on results received, patients may erroneously alter their screening habits or their lifestyles on the misconception that they have a reduced risk than previously perceived.

Arguments for DTC include the possibility of identifying unknown disease risk so increased surveillance can be undertaken. It also allows people with no risk factors the ability to access services otherwise denied to them by medical professions based on family history or well-established criteria. These consumers may feel an ability to make an autonomous decision without the paternalism of the medical community.

After weighing these issues, Wasson and colleagues[71] argue that the harm outweighs the benefits to the consumers, but contends that legislation for DTC may not be forthcoming. They make suggestions to increase the awareness and education in the medical community in regard to this type of testing and contemplate a more active role for medical geneticists to work with the DTC companies to help address the ethical concerns.

The NSGC recommends that consumers question the DTC company on several issues, including (1) accreditation; (2) compliance with the genetic testing policies set forth by professional genetic organizations (NSGC, ASHG); (3) the availability of material that addresses the clinical implications of the test and the informed consent process with assurance that the material was designed or reviewed by a professional genetic specialist; (4) recommendations regarding disclosing results to family members or health care provider; (5) availability of support from genetics experts; (6) psychologic support if needed; and (7) safeguards in regard to patient and privacy. The NSGC cautions against the use of DTC companies that cannot appropriately address the previously mentioned questions, and encourages the involvement of a clinically trained genetic professional for individuals undergoing genetic testing.[72]

SUMMARY

By gaining a better understanding of the complex ethical, legal, and psychosocial issues surrounding genetic testing for inherited CRC syndromes, the counselor is better able to explore factors that are likely to motivate, deter, and cause distress in probands who wish to undergo genetic testing. Exploring these issues, assessing the risk in the family, and relaying the necessary information about the genetic syndrome and testing process provides the tools to allow the proband to make an informed decision about genetic testing and enables the genetic counselor to best facilitate this process.

REFERENCES

1. Resta R, Biesecker B, Bennett R, et al. A new definition of genetic counseling: National Society of Genetic Counselors' task force report. J Genet Couns 2006; 15(2):77–83.
2. Lynch PM. New issues in genetic counseling of hereditary colon cancer. Clin Cancer Res 2007;13(22):6857–61.
3. Trepanier A, Ahrens M, McKinnon W, et al. Genetic cancer risk assessment and counseling: recommendations of the National Society of Genetic Counselors. J Genet Couns 2004;13(2):83–114.
4. Brain K, Sivell S, Bennert K, et al. An exploratory comparison of genetic counseling protocols for HNPCC predictive testing. Clin Genet 2005;68:255–61.

5. Aktan-Collan K, Mecklin J-P, de la Chapelle A, et al. Evaluation of a counselling protocol for predictive genetic testing for hereditary non-polyposis colorectal cancer. J Med Genet 2000;37:108–13.
6. Wakefield CE, Meiser B, Homewood J, et al. Randomized trial of a decision aid for individuals considering genetic testing for hereditary nonpolyposis colorectal cancer risk. Cancer 2008;133(5):956–65.
7. Ivanovich J, Babb S, Goodfellow P, et al. Evaluation of the family history collection process and the accuracy of cancer reporting among a series of women with endometrial cancer. Clin Cancer Res 2002;8:1849–56.
8. Soegaard M, Jensen A, Frederiksen K, et al. Accuracy of self-reported family history of cancer in a large case-control study of ovarian cancer. Cancer Causes Control 2008;19(5):469–70.
9. Mitchell RJ, Brewster D, Campbell H, et al. Accuracy of reporting of family history of colorectal cancer. Gut 2004;53:291–5.
10. Glanz K, Grove J, Le ML, et al. Underreporting of family history of colon cancer: correlates and implications. Cancer Epidemiol Biomarkers Prev 1999;8:635–9.
11. Gaff CL, Rogers MT, Frayling IM. Genetic counseling and consent for tumour testing in HNPCC. Clin Genet 2007;71:400–5.
12. Chan-Smutko G, Patel D, Shannon KM, et al. Professional challenges in cancer genetic testing: who is the patient? Oncologist 2008;13:232–8.
13. Carlsson C, Nilbert M. Living with hereditary non-polyposis cancer, experiences from and impact of genetic testing. J Genet Couns 2007;16(6):811–20.
14. Esplen MJ, Urquhart C, Butler K, et al. The experience of loss and anticipation of distress in colorectal cancer patients undergoing genetic testing. J Psychosom Res 2003;55(5):427–35.
15. Keller M, Jost R, Haunstetter CM, et al. Psychosocial outcome following genetic risk counselling for familial colorectal cancer: a comparison of affected patients and family members. Clin Genet 2008;74:414–24.
16. McAllister M. Personal theories of inheritance, coping strategies, risk perception and engagement in hereditary non-polyposis colon cancer families offered genetic testing. Clin Genet 2003;64(3):179–89.
17. Hadley DW, Jenkins J, Diamond E, et al. Genetic counseling and testing in families with hereditary nonpolyposis colorectal cancer. Arch Intern Med 2003;163: 573–82.
18. Ceballos RM, Newcomb PA, Beasley JM, et al. Colorectal cancer cases and relatives of cases indicate similar willingness to receive and disclose genetic information. Genet Test 2008;12(3):415–20.
19. Keller M, Jost R, Kadmon M. Acceptance of and attitude toward genetic testing for hereditary nonpolyposis colorectal cancer: a comparison of participants and nonparticipants in genetic counseling. Dis Colon Rectum 2004;47:153–62.
20. Lerman C, Hughes C, Trock BJ. Genetic testing in families with hereditary nonpolyposis colon cancer. JAMA 1999;281(17):1618–22.
21. Esplen MJ, Madlensky L, Aronson M, et al. Colorectal cancer survivors undergoing genetic testing for hereditary non-polyposis colorectal cancer: motivational factors and psychosocial functioning. Clin Genet 2007;72:394–401.
22. Aktan-Collan K, Mecklin JP, Jarvinen H, et al. Predictive genetic testing for hereditary non-polyposis colorectal cancer: uptake and long-term satisfaction. Int J Cancer 2000;89(1):44–50.
23. Codori AM, Petersen GM, Miglioretti DL. Attitudes toward colon cancer gene testing: factors predicting test uptake. Cancer Epidemiol Biomarkers Prev 1999;8(4 Pt 2):345–51.

24. McCann S, Macauley D, Barnett Y, et al. Family communication, genetic testing and colonoscopy screening in hereditary non-polyposis colon cancer: a qualitative study. Psychooncology 2009 [Epub ahead of print].
25. U.S. Department of Health & Human Services. Genetic Information Nondiscrimination Act of 2008. Available at: http://frwebgate.access.gpo.gov/cgi-bin/getdoc.cgi?dbname=110_cong_public_laws&docid=f:publ233.110.pdf. Accessed January 21, 2009.
26. Andrews L, Mireskandari S, Jessen J, et al. Impact of familial adenomatous polyposis on young adults: attitudes toward genetic testing, support, and information needs. Genet Med 2006;8:697–703.
27. Aktan-Collan K, Haukkala A, Mecklin J-P, et al. Psychological consequences of predictive genetic testing for hereditary non-polyposis colorectal cancer (HNPCC): a prospective follow-up study. Int J Cancer 2001;93:608–11.
28. Esplen MJ, Madlensky L, Butler K, et al. Motivations and psychosocial impact of genetic testing for HNPCC. Am J Med Genet 2001;103(1):9–15.
29. Meiser B, Collins V, Warren R, et al. Psychological impact of genetic testing for hereditary non-polyposis colorectal cancer. Clin Genet 2004;66:502–11.
30. Shiloh S, Koehly L, Jenkins J, et al. Monitoring coping style moderates emotional reactions to genetic testing for hereditary nonpolyposis colorectal cancer: a longitudinal study. Psychooncology 2008;17(8):746–55.
31. Gritz E, Peterson S, Vernon S, et al. Psychological impact of genetic testing for hereditary non-polyposis colorectal cancer. J Clin Oncol 2005;23(9):1902–10.
32. Douma KF, Aaronson NK, Vason HFA, et al. Psychosocial issues in genetic testing for familial adenomatous polyposis: a review of the literature. Psychooncology 2008;17:737–45.
33. Duncan RE, Gillam L, Savulescu J, et al. You're one of us now: young people describe their experiences of predictive genetic testing for Huntington disease (HD) and familial adenomatous polyposis (FAP). Am J Med Genet C Semin Med Genet 2008;148C:47–55.
34. Andrews L, Mireskandari S, Jessen J, et al. Impact of familial adenomatous polyposis on young adults: quality of life outcomes. Dis Colon Rectum 2007;50:1306–15.
35. Michie S, Bobrow M, Marteau TM. Predictive genetic testing in children and adults: a study of emotional impact. J Med Genet 2001;38:519–26.
36. Esplen MJ, Berk T, Butler K, et al. Quality of life in adults diagnosed with familial adenomatous polyposis and desmoids tumour. Dis Colon Rectum 2004;47:687–96.
37. American Society of Clinical Oncology policy statement update. Genetic testing for cancer susceptibility. J Clin Orthod 2003;21(12):2397–406.
38. Borry P, Goffin T, Nys H, et al. Attitudes regarding predictive genetic testing in minors: a survey of European clinical geneticist. Am J Med Genet C Semin Med Genet 2008;148C:78–83.
39. Borry P, Stultiens L, Nys H, et al. Presymptomatic and predictive genetic testing in minors: a systematic review of guidelines and position papers. Clin Genet 2006;70:374–81.
40. Whitelaw S, Northover JM, Hodgson SV. Attitudes to predictive DNA testing in familial adenomatous polyposis. J Med Genet 1996;33:540–3.
41. Codori AM, Petersen GM, Boyd PA, et al. Genetic testing for cancer in children: short-term psychological effect. Arch Pediatr Adolesc Med 1996;150:1131–8.
42. Codori AM, Zawacki KL, Petersen GM, et al. Genetic testing for hereditary colorectal cancer in children: long-term psychological effects. Am J Med Genet 2003;116A:117–28.

43. Kastrinos F, Stoffel E, Balmana J, et al. Attitudes toward prenatal genetic testing in patients with familial adenomatous polyposis. Am J Gastroenterol 2007;102: 1284–90.
44. Woo A, Sadana A, Mauger DT, et al. Psychosocial impact of Peutz-Jeghers syndrome. Fam Cancer 2009;8:59–65.
45. Offit K, Sagi M, Hurley K. Preimplantation genetic diagnosis for cancer syndromes: a new challenge for preventative medicine. JAMA 2006;296(22): 2727–30.
46. Offit K, Kohut K, Clagett B, et al. Cancer genetic testing and assisted reproduction. J Clin Oncol 2006;24(29):4775–82.
47. Rechitsky S, Verlinsky O, Chistokhina A, et al. Preimplanation genetic diagnosis for cancer predisposition. Roprod Riomed Online 2002;5:148–55.
48. Kohut K, Manno M, Gallinger S, et al. Should healthcare providers have a duty to warn family members of individuals with an HNPCC-causing mutations? A survey of patients from the Ontario Familial Colon Cancer Registry. J Med Genet 2007; 44(6):404–7.
49. Pentz RD, Peterson SK, Watts B, et al. Hereditary nonpolyposis colorectal cancer family members' perceptions about the duty to inform and health professionals' role in disseminating genetic information. Genet Test 2005;9:261–8.
50. Stoffel E, Ford B, Mercado R, et al. Sharing genetic test results in Lynch syndrome: communication with close and distant relatives. Clin Gastroenterol Hepatol 2008;6:333–8.
51. Mesters I, Ausems M, Eichhorn S, et al. Informing one's family about genetic testing for hereditary non-polyposis colorectal cancer (HNPCC): a retrospective exploratory study. Fam Cancer 2005;4(2):163–7.
52. Falk MJ, Dugan B, O'Riordan MA, et al. Medical geneticists' duty to warn at-risk relatives for genetic disease. Am J Med Genet 2003;120A:374–80.
53. Wolff K, Brun W, Kvale G, et al. Confidentiality versus duty to inform-an empirical study on attitudes towards the handling of genetic information. Am J Med Genet A 2007;143(2):142–8.
54. Peterson SK, Watts BG, Koehly LM, et al. How families communicate about HNPCC genetic testing: findings from a qualitative study. Am J Med Genet C Semin Med Genet 2003;119:78–86.
55. Aktan-Collan K, Haukkala A, Pylvänäinen K, et al. Direct contact in inviting high-risk members of hereditary colon cancer families to genetic counselling and DNA testing. J Med Genet 2007;44:732–8.
56. Pate v Threlkel, 661 So 2d 278 (Fla 1995).
57. Safer v Estate of T. Pack, 677 A 2d 1188 (NJ Supp 1996).
58. National Society of Genetic Counselors (adopted 1991; revised 2002). National Society of Genetic Counselor's position statement on confidentiality of test results. Available at: http://www.nsgc.org/about/position.cfm#Confidentiality.
59. American Medical Association. Policy statement E-2.131 disclosure of familial risk in genetic testing 2008. Available at: http://www.ama-assn.org/ama1/pub/upload/mm/31/ethicspolicies073108.pdf. Accessed January 24, 2009.
60. Gold J. To warn or not to warn? Genetic information, families and physician liability. Mcgill J Med 2004;8:72–8.
61. Lacroix M, Nycum G, Godard B, et al. Should physicians warn patients' relatives of genetic risks? CMAJ 2008;178(5):593–5.
62. Canadian Medical Association. Code of ethics of the Canadian Medical Association [Last revision, 2004]. Available at: http://policybase.cma.ca/PolicyPDF/PD04-06.pdf. Accessed January 24, 2009.

63. The American Society of Human Genetics Social Issues Subcommittee on Familial Disclosure. ASHG statement: professional disclosure of familial genetic information. Am J Hum Genet 1998;62:474–83.

64. U.S. Department of Health & Human Services. The Health Insurance Portability and Accountability Act of 1996 (HIPAA) Privacy Rule. Available at: http://www.hhs.gov/ocr/privacy/index.html. Accessed January 21, 2009.

65. Personal Health Information Protection Act and Quality of Care Information Protection Act (November 2004). Available at: http://www.health.gov.on.ca/english/providers/legislation/priv_legislation/priv_legislation.html. Accessed January 24, 2009.

66. Offit K, Groeger E, Turner S, et al. The duty to warn a patient's family members about hereditary disease risks. JAMA 2004;292:1469–73.

67. Forrest LE, Delatycki MB, Skene L, et al. Communicating genetic information in families: a review of guidelines and positive papers. Eur J Hum Genet 2007;15:612–8.

68. Godard B, Hurlimann T, Letendre M, et al. Guidelines for disclosing genetic information to family members: from development to use. Fam Cancer 2006;5(1):103–16.

69. Dugan RB, Wiesner GL, Juengst ET, et al. Duty to warn at-risk relatives for genetic disease: genetic counselors' clinical experience. Am J Med Genet C Semin Med Genet 2003;119C:27–34.

70. Schneider KA, Chittenden AB, Branda KJ, et al. Ethical issues in cancer genetics: I1 whose information is it? J Genet Couns 2006;15(6):491–503.

71. Wasson K, Cook ED, Helzlsouer K. Direct-to-consumer online genetic testing and the four principles: an analysis of the ethical issues. Ethics Med 2006;22(2):83–91.

72. National Society of Genetic Counselors position statement on direct-to-consumer genetic testing (adopted 2007). Available at: http://www.nsgc.org/about/position.cfm%23DTC%5D.

Genetic Testing for Hereditary Colorectal Cancer

Heather Hampel, MS, CGC

KEYWORDS

- Genetic • Testing • Lynch syndrome • Polyposis syndromes
- Colorectal neoplasm

Genetic testing for hereditary colorectal cancer syndromes is more complex than genetic testing for hereditary breast-ovarian cancer syndrome. This complexity is due to the following: (1) there are many more syndromes to consider in the differential diagnosis; (2) some of the syndromes have considerable phenotypic overlap; (3) many of the syndromes can be caused by mutations in any one of several causative genes; and (4) testing for Lynch syndrome (the most common hereditary cause of colorectal cancer) includes a combination of tumor testing and germline genetic testing. As a result, many clinicians find genetic testing for hereditary colorectal cancer to be a challenge. The clinical features of all the various hereditary colorectal cancer syndromes have been reviewed in other articles in this issue. In addition, genetic counseling, which is a prerequisite for genetic testing to ensure appropriate informed consent, has been reviewed by Melyssa Aronson. This article focuses on genetic testing for hereditary colorectal cancer syndromes.

The hereditary colorectal cancer syndromes can be divided into the polyposis and nonpolyposis syndromes, keeping in mind that there are polyps in the nonpolyposis syndromes; however, they are usually less numerous. The presence of ten colonic polyps is sometimes used as a rough threshold for when to consider genetic testing for a polyposis syndrome. The polyposis syndromes can be further subdivided by the histology of the polyps, namely the hamartomatous and adenomatous polyposis syndromes. Hamartomatous polyposis syndromes include juvenile polyposis syndrome (JPS), Peutz-Jeghers syndrome (PJS), hyperplastic polyposis syndrome (HPS), and the *PTEN* hamartomatous tumor syndrome (PHTS; comprised of Cowden syndrome [CS] and Bannayan-Ruvalcaba-Riley [BRR] syndrome). Adenomatous polyposis syndromes include familial adenomatous polyposis (FAP), attenuated FAP (AFAP), and *MUTYH*-associated polyposis (MAP). A diagnosis of mixed polyposis syndrome should be considered in individuals with both hamartomatous and

---

Division of Human Genetics, Department of Internal Medicine, The Ohio State University Comprehensive Cancer Center, 2001 Polaris Parkway, Columbus, OH 43240, USA
E-mail address: Heather.Hampel@osumc.edu

Surg Oncol Clin N Am 18 (2009) 687–703
doi:10.1016/j.soc.2009.08.001
surgonc.theclinics.com

adenomatous colon polyps and with no features of the other polyposis syndromes. The nonpolyposis syndromes include Lynch syndrome (LS), familial colorectal cancer syndrome type X, and occasionally can include individuals with MAP and a low polyp count. A flowchart demonstrating this differential diagnosis is shown in **Fig. 1**.

Genetic testing is now available on a clinical basis for every gene discussed in this article. To find a list of laboratories performing genetic testing for any of these genes, visit the GeneTests Web site at www.genetests.org. When selecting a laboratory for clinical testing, there are many factors to consider. Whereas price and billing considerations may be the paramount concern to the patient, it is also very important to consider the testing modality used (sequencing versus other mutation screening modalities and whether testing for large rearrangements is included), as this can significantly affect the sensitivity of the test. The importance of including large rearrangement testing varies from gene to gene, and is discussed throughout this article.

GENETIC TESTING FOR THE POLYPOSIS SYNDROMES

Genetic testing for the polyposis syndromes is generally more straightforward than testing for the nonpolyposis syndromes; however, several of the conditions are polygenic, and genetic testing does not have 100% sensitivity for any of the syndromes at this time. As such, the most important prerequisite for genetic testing in the polyposis syndromes is making certain of the differential diagnosis to select the correct gene test. To that end, it is often recommended that a dedicated gastrointestinal pathologist review the pathology of the polyps to confirm the type of polyp when there is any

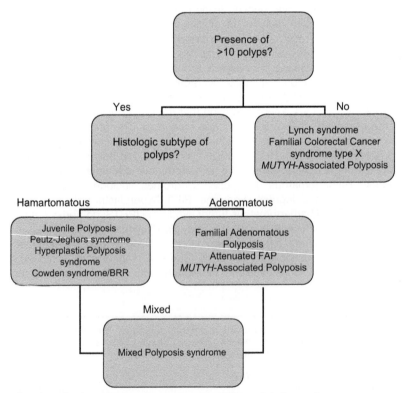

Fig. 1. Flowchart for hereditary colorectal cancer differential diagnosis.

doubt. Once the syndrome has been correctly identified, testing should proceed as described here.

HAMARTOMATOUS POLYPOSIS SYNDROMES
Juvenile Polyposis Syndrome

JPS (Online Mendelian Inheritance in Man [OMIM] 174900) can be due to mutations in either the BMPR1A gene or the SMAD4 gene. SMAD4 is located on chromosome 18q21.1 and was identified as a susceptibility gene for JPS in 1998.[1] BMPR1A is located on chromosome 10q22.3 and was identified as the second gene responsible for JPS in 2001.[2] Data from all studies involving sequencing and large rearrangement testing (using multiplex ligation-dependent probe assay, or MLPA) of these genes in JPS patients were reviewed recently.[3] Point mutations were found in 40.1% of JPS patients; this included 21.6% (77/357) with SMAD4 mutations and 18.5% (62/336) with BMPR1A mutations. Large rearrangements were found in 8.7% of JPS patients; this included 4.6% (9/194) with SMAD4 deletions and 4.1% (8/194) with BMPR1A deletions. The likelihood of finding a SMAD4 mutation (26.8%) was approximately the same as the likelihood of finding a BMPR1A mutation (23.7%) when the analysis was restricted to only the 3 studies that included both sequencing and MLPA. Although the likelihood of finding a mutation in either gene is about equal, testing could still be ordered one gene at a time to potentially save the patient money (because the second gene test would not be necessary if a mutation was found in the first gene). Due to the association of SMAD4 mutations with hereditary hemorrhagic telangiectasia, mutations in this gene are more likely if a patient with JPS reports a history of recurrent nosebleeds, arteriovenous malformations, or telangiectasias.[4] Unfortunately, the causative mutation will only be identified in around 50% of patients with a clinical diagnosis of JPS when genetic testing includes both sequencing and MLPA of the SMAD4 and BMPR1A genes. This situation suggests that there are possibly additional genes that cause JPS or other mutations that inactivate SMAD4 and BMPR1A that cannot be detected currently. Such a situation also means that a negative genetic test result for SMAD4 and BMPR1A will not rule out the diagnosis of JPS, and cannot be used to exclude the diagnosis in a patient who does not meet the clinical diagnostic criteria for JPS.

Peutz-Jeghers Syndrome

PJS (OMIM 175200) is caused by mutations in the STK11 gene (also known as LKB1). STK11 is located on chromosome 19p13.3, and mutations in this gene were found to cause PJS in 1998.[5] Combining data from the 2 largest series of PJS patients tested for mutations in STK11 by full sequencing and MLPA yields the following results.[5,6] Out of 132 patients meeting the clinical diagnostic criteria for PJS, mutations were identified in 85% (112/132); this includes 84 (63.6%) point mutations identified by sequencing and 28 (21.2%) large deletions identified by MLPA. These results make it less likely that there is another as yet unidentified gene for PJS; however, there are some linkage studies in PJS families that have reported exclusion of the STK11 locus.[7-9] At this point, a negative test result cannot rule out a diagnosis of PJS but mutations will be identified in the majority of patients with a clinical diagnosis of PJS if testing includes both sequencing and large rearrangement analysis of the STK11 gene.

Hyperplastic Polyposis Syndrome

The gene(s) responsible for HPS (not included in OMIM) have not been identified. Clinicians should try to enroll patients meeting a clinical diagnosis of HPS into a research study attempting to identify the responsible gene. In the meantime, the diagnosis can only be made clinically based on the World Health Organization diagnostic criteria; 5 or more hyperplastic polyps proximal to the sigmoid colon with 2 measuring greater than 1 cm in diameter, or more than 30 hyperplastic polyps anywhere in the colon.[10]

PTEN Hamartoma Tumor Syndrome

PHTS includes syndromes caused by germline mutations in the PTEN gene, including CS (OMIM 158350) and BRR syndrome (OMIM 153480). The PTEN gene is located on chromosome 10q23.3, and mutations in this gene were associated with CS and BRR syndrome in 1997.[11,12] A recent review[13] found that there is not strong evidence of an increased risk for colorectal cancer among patients with PHTS; however, it is likely that 70% to 80% of patients with PHTS have colon polyps when they are evaluated with colonoscopy.[14–16] Although it is generally stated that 80% of CS patients will have PTEN mutations, by combining the published findings of 5 studies that included sequencing of the PTEN gene in patients meeting the diagnostic criteria for CS, it seems that a mutation will be identified only 53% (54/101) of the time.[11,17–19] Large deletions seem to be rare in this gene, with 2 studies reporting a combined prevalence of 2.3% (4/175) among CS or CS-like patients without identifiable point mutations in the PTEN gene.[20,21] Variations in the promoter region have been reported in 10% (9/95) of patients who are negative for a PTEN mutation on sequencing (around 2% of all CS patients); however, it is not yet clear whether these mutations are deleterious.[20] PTEN gene sequencing seems to be sufficient at present for PTEN testing in a patient suspected of having PHTS, because the addition of large deletion or promoter mutation analysis will only add 2% to 3% to the overall mutation detection rate. This finding may indicate that there are other genes responsible for some cases of CS, other changes that inactivate the PTEN gene that cannot be detected at present, or possibly that the diagnostic criteria are not stringent enough given that many of the features of this syndrome (fibrocystic breasts, thyroid nodules, endometrial fibroids) are common in the general population. A negative result cannot rule out the diagnosis, given the low detection rate at this time.

ADENOMATOUS POLYPOSIS SYNDROMES

Because there is considerable overlap among the adenomatous polyposis syndromes, the approaches to genetic testing for all 3 syndromes are described at the end of the following 3 sections.

Familial Adenomatous Polyposis

FAP (OMIM 175100) is caused by mutations in the APC gene located on chromosome 5q21-22. Mutations in the APC gene were determined to cause FAP in 1991.[22,23] Genetic testing for APC mutations has changed significantly over the past 10 years. In the late 1990s the only APC testing available clinically in the United States was protein truncation testing. This type of test was followed by full sequencing of the APC gene, and then large rearrangement analysis (using an approach like MLPA). Depending on the clinical features present in the patient and the testing modality used (single-strand conformation polymorphism [SSCP], denaturing gradient gel electrophoresis [DGGE], or protein truncation testing [PTT] were used in most studies), mutations in the APC gene are found in 48% to 80% of patients with polyposis.[24–26] In the largest study to date involving 680 polyposis families, APC mutations were found in 31.7% of patients with less than 100 adenomas and 58.2% of patients with more than 100 adenomas.[24] The addition of large rearrangement testing of the *APC* gene has been shown to detect mutations in an additional 4% to 33% of polyposis patients who had previously tested negative.[27-31] Therefore, *APC* gene testing should always include both testing for point mutations (using sequencing or another technique) and large rearrangement analysis. In addition, since 2002 it has been shown that 7.5% to 17% of classic polyposis patients have biallelic *MUTYH* mutations. As a result, for patients who previously tested negative for *APC* mutations, there may be additional testing available that could help identify the cause of their polyposis.[32]

Attenuated FAP

AFAP (OMIM 175100) is described in patients with 10 to 99 adenomas. AFAP can be caused either by germline mutations in the *APC* gene (discussed earlier) or by biallelic mutations in the *MUTYH* gene (described later). In a series of 25 Dutch families who met AFAP criteria,[33] *APC* mutations were found in 9 families (36%) and biallelic *MUTYH* mutations were found in 9 families (36%). There was no significant difference in the clinical features of the families with *APC* or *MUTYH* mutations. Despite the fact that the *APC* mutations responsible for AFAP tend to occur at either the 5' end of the gene (the first 5 exons), in exon 9, or at the distal 3' end of the gene,[34] full gene sequencing is necessary, because exceptions have been reported and there is no targeted *APC* test available for AFAP.

MUTYH-Associated Polyposis

MAP (OMIM 608456) is caused by biallelic mutations in the *MUTYH* gene. MAP is the only known example of an autosomal recessive colon cancer susceptibility syndrome. The *MUTYH* gene is located on chromosome 1p32.1, and was found to cause polyposis and colon cancer in 2002.[35] The presentation is variable; most patients have attenuated polyposis but some have classic polyposis indistinguishable from FAP and others have colon cancer without polyposis (leading to clinical overlap with LS). A recent review[32] found that 5% to 22% of patients with 3 to 100 adenomas and 7.5% to 17% of patients with more than 100 adenomas have biallelic *MUTYH* mutations.[36-40] Most of the mutations found in the *MUTYH* gene have been missense mutations. The 2 most common *MUTYH* mutations are the Y179C (previously known as Y165C before a nomenclature change) and G396D (previously known as G382D before a nomenclature change) mutations, which account for 73% of *MUTYH* mutations found in Caucasian populations with Northern European ancestry.[41] Other *MUTYH* mutations seen commonly include the R245C and IVS10-2a>g mutations in Japanese MAP patients, the c.1145delC mutation in Italian MAP patients, A473D in Finnish MAP patients, and E383fxX451 found in Portuguese MAP patients.[32]

Given the recessive inheritance pattern, siblings of an affected individual are at the highest risk for also having biallelic *MUTYH* mutations (25% risk) and should be offered genetic testing. In addition, testing should be offered to the spouse of a biallelic mutation carrier if there are at-risk children in the family because of the relatively high carrier frequency (2% in North America).[42] If the spouse does not have a *MUTYH* mutation, then the children will all be carriers and should be aware of the future risk to their offspring (should they have children with a carrier), but none of them will have MAP due to biallelic mutations. If the spouse does have a *MUTYH* mutation, then the children will each have a 50% chance of being a biallelic mutation carrier and having MAP. This condition can create a "pseudodominant" inheritance pattern because the parent and 50% of the children will be affected with MAP.

GENETIC TESTING FOR FAMILIAL ADENOMATOUS POLYPOSIS, ATTENUATED FAMILIAL ADENOMATOUS POLYPOSIS, AND *MUTYH*-ASSOCIATED POLYPOSIS

It is often not easy to distinguish FAP patients (due to *APC* mutations) from MAP patients, given (1) the high de novo mutation rate of *APC* mutations (leading to single affected individuals), (2) the high carrier rate of *MUTYH* mutations (leading to pseudo-dominant inheritance), and (3) that FAP-associated extracolonic features (congenital hypertrophy of the retinal pigment epithelium, upper gastrointestinal polyps, and desmoid tumors) have occasionally been reported in MAP patients.[32] Genetic testing for patients with more than 10 adenomatous polyps should include testing for both the *APC* gene and the *MUTYH* gene. Such testing is particularly important to the family members of polyposis patients because the inheritance pattern of *APC* (autosomal dominant) and *MUTYH* (autosomal recessive) differ, and this significantly affects the risks to the children and siblings of affected individuals.

If a family appears to have a vertical transmission pattern of polyposis (ie, affected individuals in more than one generation), genetic testing should begin with *APC*. If negative, testing should proceed to *MUTYH* despite the vertical transmission pattern, given the possibility of pseudodominant inheritance. Practically speaking, a combination test including *APC* testing and screening for the 2 most common *MUTYH* mutations is available and is often a good approach for patients with adenomatous polyps. *APC* testing should always include testing for point mutations and large rearrangements to maximize mutation detection. In North America, *MUTYH* genetic testing often begins with the Y179C and G396D mutations, and proceeds to full sequencing if the patient is found to be heterozygous for 1 of these 2 mutations. The concern with this approach is that it will miss those patients who carry 2 *MUTYH* mutations other than Y179C or G396D. Studies have found that 8.3% to 20% of polyposis patients with biallelic *MUTYH* mutations identified through full sequencing did not have either of the 2 common mutations.[36,42,43] As a result, it is appropriate and cost-effective to begin testing with the *APC* gene and the 2 common *MUTYH* mutations in Caucasian polyposis patients with Northern European ancestry. However, full sequencing of the *MUTYH* gene is indicated if no mutations are found in *APC* or in the initial *MUTYH* 2 mutation screening test. Full sequencing of the *MUTYH* gene (instead of the 2 mutation screen) would be more appropriate for anyone who is not Caucasian with Northern European ancestry.

HEREDITARY MIXED POLYPOSIS SYNDROME

The gene(s) responsible for hereditary mixed polyposis syndrome (HMPS) (OMIM 601228 and 610069) have not been identified at this time, although there is linkage to the CRAC1 locus on chromosome 15q13-14 among Ashkenazi Jewish patients.[44–46] Linkage to chromosome 10q23 was found in 2 Singapore Chinese families, and one was found to have a *BMPR1A* gene mutation.[47] As a result, clinicians should try to enroll patients meeting a clinical diagnosis of mixed polyposis syndrome into a research study attempting to identify the responsible gene(s). Patients with HMPS have a combination of juvenile, hyperplastic, and adenomatous polyps, causing this to be a diagnosis of exclusion after the known genes for other polyposis syndromes have been ruled out.

NONPOLYPOSIS SYNDROMES

The most common hereditary colorectal cancer syndrome is LS, and this accounts for most cases of the hereditary nonpolyposis colorectal cancers. As a result, this syndrome needs to be ruled out by tumor testing before consideration of the other possible syndromes within this category.

Lynch Syndrome

LS (OMIM 120435) is the most common hereditary cause of colorectal cancer, accounting for around 3% of all cases.[48,49] LS can be caused by mutations in any 1 of at least 4 mismatch repair genes: *MLH1* (chromosome 3p21.3), *MSH2* (chromosome 2p22-21), *MSH6* (chromosome 2p16), and *PMS2* (chromosome 7p22.2). Testing for LS is more complicated than testing for most other hereditary cancer syndromes, because of the genetic heterogeneity and because there are 2 screening tests that can be performed on tumor material from the patients before gene testing. The tumor screening tests include microsatellite instability testing and immunohistochemistry staining for the 4 mismatch repair proteins.

MICROSATELLITE INSTABILITY

Microsatellites are repetitive DNA sequences (usually a lengthy repeat of 1 to 2 nucleotides) that occur throughout the genome. These areas are prone to an increase or decrease in the number of repeats when the mismatch repair genes are not functioning properly. This change occurs in the tumor DNA from LS patients, and is known as microsatellite instability (MSI).[50–52] MSI testing assesses the length of 5 microsatellites or more using tumor DNA and, for comparison, normal DNA.[52] MSI-high tumors are defined as tumors having changes in the length of at least 2 of the 5 (>20%) microsatellites in tumor DNA versus normal DNA. MSI-low tumors are those tumors having changes in the length of 1 of the 5 ($\leq$20%) microsatellites. Microsatellite stable (MSS) tumors have no changes in the length of the microsatellites being studied.[53]

IMMUNOHISTOCHEMICAL STAINING

Immunohistochemical staining (IHC) for the 4 mismatch repair (MMR) proteins determines whether these proteins are present in the tumor. When one or more of the MMR proteins is absent in the tumor tissue, IHC is considered abnormal.[54,55] This abnormality is an indication that the protein is not being expressed in the tumor as a result either of germline mutation or epigenetic silencing. Because genetic testing is expensive, IHC is helpful because the results can narrow down the number of MMR genes that need to be tested from all 4 to only 1 or 2. Understanding the underlying functions of the MMR proteins helps in the interpretation of IHC results. The MMR proteins are only stable when they are in heterodimer pairs.[56–59] MSH2 can pair with either MSH6 or MSH3, whereas MSH6 can only pair with MSH2.[56] As a result, if there is a germline mutation in *MSH2*, MSH6 has no partner with whom to make a heterodimer pair and the tumor generally is missing both the MSH2 and MSH6 proteins. However, if there is a germline mutation in *MSH6*, MSH2 is typically stable because it can partner with MSH3 and the tumor will generally exhibit the absence of MSH6 only and presence of MSH2 on IHC. In a similar way MLH1 can pair with PMS1, PMS2, or MLH3, whereas PMS2 can only pair with MLH1.[59,60] This process means that if there is a germline mutation (or acquired promoter methylation) of the *MLH1* gene, PMS2 is unstable because it has no partner protein with whom to pair, and both MLH1 and PMS2 will be absent in the tumor. If there is a germline mutation in *PMS2*, on the other hand, *MLH1* will generally be present in the tumor because it can partner with other mismatch repair proteins.

SENSITIVITY AND SPECIFICITY OF MICROSATELLITE INSTABILITY AND IMMUNOHISTOCHEMICAL STAINING

The majority of patients whose colorectal tumors are MSI-high (75%) or have abnormal IHC (88%) do not have LS.[48,49] In these cases, the cause of the deficient mismatch repair is usually acquired hypermethylation of the MLH1 gene promoter. As a result, whereas MSI and IHC can identify colorectal cancer patients who are more likely to have LS, these tests are not diagnostic. Some argue that proceeding directly to gene testing is an acceptable approach in patients with a high likelihood of having LS (eg, families meeting the Amsterdam criteria,[61,62] or families with 5%–10% or more likelihood of having an MMR gene mutation based on current risk assessment models, MMRpredict,[63] MMRpro,[64] or PREMM1,2[65]). However, around 50% of families that meet Amsterdam I criteria do not have an identifiable MMR gene mutation, and would undergo expensive and unnecessary genetic testing with this approach.[66] In addition, ordering IHC will save money overall by reducing the number of genes that need to be tested. As a result, many argue that when possible, LS testing should always begin with MSI and IHC on an LS-associated tumor.

A recent review[67] found that the sensitivity of MSI was 89% for patients with MLH1 and MSH2 mutations, and 77% for patients with MSH6 mutations as long as at least 3 mononucleotide repeats were included in the panel of microsatellites tested. The sensitivity dropped to 80% and 84% for MLH1 and MSH2 mutation carriers, and 55% for MSH6 mutation carriers if only 2 mononucleotide repeats were included in the test. The specificity was 90.2%. The sensitivity of IHC was 83% regardless of which MMR gene was involved, and specificity was 88.8%. This review did not assess the sensitivity of using both MSI and IHC on the same tumor to screen for LS because its aim was to select 1 of the 2 screening tests for use among all newly diagnosed colorectal cancer patients. However, assuming that some of the tumors from LS patients that are missed by MSI are detected by IHC and vice versa, which has been reported,[48,49] a gain in sensitivity would be expected by the use of both tests. Therefore, when screening a patient in a high-risk clinical setting, it is advisable to order both MSI and IHC on the LS-associated tumor.

HOW TO FOLLOW UP MICROSATELLITE INSTABILITY AND IMMUNOHISTOCHEMICAL STAINING RESULTS

If the tumor is MSS and IHC indicates that all 4 MMR proteins are present, then the patient is unlikely to have LS. Genetic testing for the MMR genes would not be indicated in this case. If the family history is strong, it may be worthwhile to test a tumor from another affected family member in case the first person tested was a phenocopy (someone who happened to have an LS-associated cancer in a family with LS who did not inherit the germline MMR gene mutation segregating in the family).

If IHC indicates that one or more MMR proteins are absent (regardless of the MSI results), then the patient is more likely to have LS and genetic testing should be offered to the patient using the IHC results for guidance (**Fig. 2**). When the MSH2 and MSH6 proteins are absent, then the patient probably has LS, given the lack of evidence of other epigenetic causes for this staining pattern. MSH2 genetic testing should be ordered first, because mutations in this gene are more common among colorectal cancer patients with this IHC result. If no mutation is found in MSH2, MSH6 genetic testing should be ordered. If the MSH6 protein is the only protein absent in the tumor, then MSH6 genetic testing should be ordered. If only the PMS2 protein is absent, then PMS2 genetic testing is indicated.

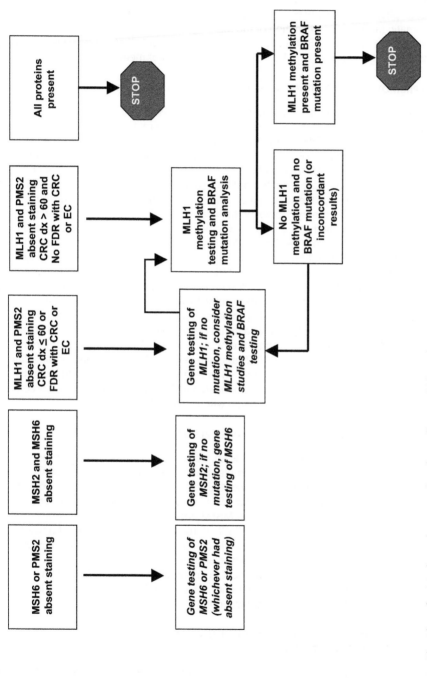

Fig. 2. Flowchart for Lynch syndrome testing depending on IHC result.

Follow-up is more complicated when the *MLH1* and *PMS2* proteins are absent in a tumor. If the patient has a strong family history, he or she may have LS due to a germline mutation in *MLH1*, and genetic testing for *MLH1* is appropriate. If the patient does not have a strong family history (perhaps they received IHC as part of routine screening at the hospital where they had surgery for their colorectal cancer), he or she probably has somatic (acquired) methylation of the *MLH1* gene promoter, but it is still possible that the patient may have LS. There are 2 tumor tests available that can help distinguish the patients with LS from the patients with *MLH1* promoter methylation.

MLH1 PROMOTER METHYLATION AND *BRAF* TESTING ON TUMOR DNA

Methylation of the *MLH1* gene promoter can be assessed directly in tumor DNA. In addition, tumors can be studied for somatic *BRAF* gene mutations (most commonly the V600E mutation). *BRAF* mutations are identified in 69% of colorectal tumors from individuals with *MLH1* promoter methylation and thus far, have not been reported in patients with germline *MLH1* mutations.[67] *BRAF* testing is not informative for endometrial tumors. Tumors found to have both *MLH1* promoter methylation and a *BRAF* mutation are most likely due to acquired *MLH1* promoter methylation, and genetic testing for LS is not necessary. However, tumors found to have *MLH1* promoter methylation and *BRAF* results that are not concordant could still be the result of a germline *MLH1* mutation, and genetic testing for *MLH1* is appropriate. *MLH1* promoter methylation without a *BRAF* mutation might occur if the *MLH1* methylation was the "second hit" in a patient with a germline *MLH1* mutation. A *BRAF* mutation might be found in a tumor from a patient with a germline *MLH1* mutation (without *MLH1* promoter methylation in the tumor) because it is unlikely that *BRAF* testing will be 100% specific. Colorectal cancer patients with *MLH1* promoter methylation are generally diagnosed at later ages, and are less likely to have a family history of colon cancer. As such, it may be prudent to order *MLH1* promoter methylation and *BRAF* testing for colorectal cancer patients with *MLH1* and *PMS2* absence on IHC if they are diagnosed after age 60 years and have no first-degree relatives with colorectal or endometrial cancer. If they are younger than 60 at diagnosis or have a first-degree relative with colorectal or endometrial cancer, testing could begin with the *MLH1* gene.

UNEXPECTED IMMUNOHISTOCHEMICAL STAINING RESULTS

The IHC results will occasionally be confusing, based on the known heterodimer pairs that occur with MMR proteins. For example, Baudhuin and colleagues[68] found that *MLH1* and *MSH6* were absent in around 1% to 3% of colon tumors studied, and *MSH6* and *PMS2* were absent in less than 1% of colon tumors. There are mononucleotide repeats in the coding region of the *MSH2*, *MSH6* and *PMS2* genes which can become unstable in an MSI-high tumor.[69] When this occurs, it can create a frameshift resulting in premature truncation of one allele of the gene. Because something would have to destroy the function of the both alleles of the same gene to result in the absence of the protein in the tumor, this occurs rarely. It has been noted that this probably occurs in subclones of an MSI-high tumor, which could also explain partial loss of IHC staining in some tumors (ie, focal staining).[70]

MICROSATELLITE INSTABILITY-HIGH TUMORS WITH NORMAL IMMUNOHISTOCHEMICAL STAINING RESULTS

A tumor will occasionally be found to be MSI-high, but the presence of all 4 MMR proteins will be demonstrated by IHC. This finding is more likely in the case of a germline missense mutation, which might lead to a full-length protein that is nonfunctional but present in the tumor, and stable in its heterodimer pair. These results can be followed up in 2 ways depending on the *a priori* likelihood that the patient has LS. One option is to order *MLH1* methylation or *BRAF* mutation testing on the colorectal tumor. Results of the *MLH1* methylation and *BRAF* mutation testing should be interpreted as described previously; this is a good option if there is not a strong family history. The second option is to proceed directly to genetic testing using a blood sample from the patient. In this case, genetic testing should start with the *MLH1* and *MSH2* genes because they are the most common causes of LS, accounting for 70% of cases.[67] If negative, proceed to *MSH6* testing and *PMS2* testing in any sequence, because these genes each account for around 15% of LS.[67]

LYNCH SYNDROME GENE TESTING

Gene testing for all 4 mismatch repair genes should include both full sequencing of the gene and large rearrangement testing, because large deletions account for around 22% of *MLH1* and *PMS2* mutations, 26% of *MSH2* mutations, and 7% of *MSH6* mutations.[48,49,71,72] Deleterious mutations in any of the 4 mismatch repair genes are diagnostic for LS. Variants of uncertain significance are found fairly frequently ($\sim$7%) in the mismatch repair genes.[48,49] For more information about a variant, one can contact the testing laboratory, conduct additional segregation testing in the family, and for variants in *MLH1* and *MSH2* use the MAPP-MMR program (http://mappmmr.blueankh.com) to find out if the mutation is likely to be deleterious or a benign polymorphism.[73] Until the pathogenicity of the mutation has been established, predictive testing should not be offered to at-risk relatives.

Management recommendations are complicated if IHC shows absence of *MSH2* and *MSH6*, or absence of *MSH6* or *PMS2* alone and genetic testing is negative. If *MLH1* and *PMS2* are absent on IHC, genetic testing is negative, and *MLH1* promoter methylation has been ruled out, surveillance recommendations are similarly complicated. A conservative approach would be to recommend that these families follow LS cancer surveillance guidelines, but this has to be interpreted in the context of the family history using clinical judgment.

FAMILIAL COLORECTAL CANCER SYNDROME TYPE X

For patients with a strong family history of colorectal cancer and MSS tumors, one should consider a diagnosis of familial colorectal cancer type X.[74] The strict definition includes only families that meet the Amsterdam I criteria with no evidence of deficient mismatch repair.[61] These families do not have an increased risk for the extracolonic cancers seen in LS. In addition, the colorectal cancer risk seems lower than in families with LS.[74] The gene(s) responsible for the colorectal cancer risk in these families have yet to be discovered, which is the reason they are referred to as "type X" at this time. This syndrome seems to also be inherited in an autosomal dominant manner so the children of an affected individual are at 50% risk for also having inherited the colorectal cancer susceptibility. Because clinical testing is not available, it may be useful to try to enroll these families in research studies looking for new colorectal cancer susceptibility genes. All at-risk individuals should receive increased colorectal cancer surveillance.

MUTYH-ASSOCIATED POLYPOSIS IN THE DIFFERENTIAL DIAGNOSIS
FOR NONPOLYPOSIS COLORECTAL CANCER

It is clear that patients with MAP do not always have significant numbers of colon polyps, leading to some overlap with the nonpolyposis syndromes. In addition, there are case reports of MAP patients with sebaceous adenomas or carcinomas that would be typical in the Muir-Torre variant of LS. Further underscoring the clinical overlap with Lynch syndrome, a commercial laboratory found that 1% of 306 patients who had been negative for LS genetic testing had biallelic *MUTYH* mutations.[42] Biallelic *MYH* mutations have been identified in around 0.8% to 6% of colorectal cancer patients diagnosed under age 50 years, sometimes without associated adenomatous polyps.[40,75,76] A large population-based series of 9268 colorectal cancer patients was recently tested for the common Y179C and G306D *MUTYH* mutations.[76] It was determined that biallelic mutations account for 0.3% (27/9268) of all colorectal cancers, these cancers are MSS, and biallelic mutations infer a 28-fold increased risk for colorectal cancer. Four of the 27 (14.8%) patients with biallelic *MUTYH* mutations did not have any concurrent adenomas. A review of the clinical findings of 257 patients with biallelic *MUTYH* mutations found that 20% of G396D homozygotes had fewer than 10 colon polyps, compared with only 2% of the Y179C homozygotes.[77] In general, the Y179C mutation and truncating mutations in *MUTYH* were associated with higher numbers of colon polyps. Nine percent of patients with nontruncating mutations in *MU-TYH* had fewer than 10 polyps compared with none of the patients with 2 truncating mutations. At this time, it is not clear when to perform *MUTYH* gene testing in cases with less than 10 adenomatous polyps; however, it could be considered in patients with MSS colorectal cancers diagnosed under age 50 years.

GENETIC TESTING IN FAMILY MEMBERS

Clinicians must take reasonable steps to guarantee that immediate family members are warned about their risk for inherited cancer susceptibility syndromes. There is legal precedent for this in the United States (Safer v Estate of Pack, 1996) where the daughter of a man with FAP sued the estate of her father's physician for not having warned her about her risk for inheriting FAP. The New Jersey Supreme Court ruled that clinicians have a duty to warn at risk relatives of a patient with an inherited condition even if it requires that confidentiality be breached.[78] In a similar case in Florida (Pate v Threlkel), it was found that this duty is fulfilled if the doctor informs their patient that the condition is hereditary and the patient then has the responsibility for warning their at-risk relatives.[78] There are many FAP patients who have never undergone genetic testing because it was believed that this was not important given the obvious clinical diagnosis. However, this is important to the at-risk relatives of these patients who may or may not have inherited the causative gene mutation that would significantly affect their medical management. In general, all patients with a known or suspected hereditary colorectal cancer syndrome need to be referred for genetic counseling and possibly genetic testing because of the implications to their relatives and the possible implications to their own management.

Once a deleterious mutation has been identified in any of the colorectal cancer susceptibility genes in an affected family member, at-risk relatives can undergo single mutation testing for the known mutation (or mutations in the case of *MUTYH*) in the family, which is less costly and very reliable. Genetic testing can be offered to minors for conditions that require medical management in childhood (which is the case for all the polyposis syndromes). Any relative who has the mutation(s) or who defers genetic testing should be managed as if they have the condition. Any relative who does not have the known familial mutation can follow the American Cancer Society guidelines for cancer screening in the general population as long as they do not have any other cancer risk factors.

If a deleterious mutation cannot be identified in the family, then at-risk relatives either need to screen as if they have the syndrome for which they are at risk, or follow a modified screening program that may relax over time if they do not begin to exhibit signs of the condition. For example, if a person at risk for FAP does not have adenomas by a certain age, it becomes unlikely that they inherited FAP, and they may be able to undergo colonoscopy less frequently. It is important to consider when the original genetic testing occurred in the family and what testing modality was used, because advances in technology have led to increased mutation detection rates. For example, a patient who was tested for APC mutations in 1999 may have only had PTT. If no protein truncation was detected at that time, it would be important to offer APC testing using DNA sequencing and large rearrangement analysis along with MYH gene testing, because the underlying genetic cause of their polyposis may be identified with these new tests.

SUMMARY

With the recent availability of *PMS2* genetic testing on a clinical basis, genetic testing is now available in North America for all of the known hereditary colorectal cancer genes. In addition, most of these tests have improved significantly in the past few years with the inclusion of techniques to detect large rearrangements. As a result, clinicians are in a better position than ever to help families with these syndromes to identify the underlying genetic cause. This identification will ensure that they receive appropriate management, and will enable their relatives to determine their precise risks and to tailor their cancer surveillance. Because colorectal cancer can often be prevented if surveillance is initiated at the correct age and frequency, this is important for the relatives of patients with hereditary colorectal cancer syndromes.

ACKNOWLEDGMENTS

Heather Hampel is supported by grant CA16058 from the National Cancer Institute, USA. I would like to thank Rebecca Nagy, MS, CGC, Robert Pilarski, MS, CGC, and Judith Westman, MD for critical review of the manuscript. I would also like to thank Victoria Schunemann, BS for assistance with manuscript preparation.

REFERENCES

1. Howe JR, Roth S, Ringold JC, et al. Mutations in the SMAD4/DPC4 gene in juvenile polyposis. Science 1998;280:1086.
2. Howe JR, Bair JL, Sayed MG, et al. Germline mutations of the gene encoding bone morphogenetic protein receptor 1A in juvenile polyposis. Nat Genet 2001; 28:184.
3. Calva-Cerqueira D, Chinnathambi S, Pechman B, et al. The rate of germline mutations and large deletions of SMAD4 and BMPR1A in juvenile polyposis. Clin Genet 2009;75:79.
4. Gallione CJ, Repetto GM, Legius E, et al. A combined syndrome of juvenile polyposis and hereditary haemorrhagic telangiectasia associated with mutations in MADH4 (SMAD4). Lancet 2004;363:852.
5. Hemminki A, Markie D, Tomlinson I, et al. A serine/threonine kinase gene defective in Peutz-Jeghers syndrome. Nature 1998;391:184.

6. Aretz S, Stienen D, Uhlhaas S, et al. High proportion of large genomic STK11 deletions in Peutz-Jeghers syndrome. Hum Mutat 2005;26:513.

7. Buchet-Poyau K, Mehenni H, Radhakrishna U, et al. Search for the second Peutz-Jeghers syndrome locus: exclusion of the STK13, PRKCG, KLK10, and PSCD2 genes on chromosome 19 and the STK11IP gene on chromosome 2. Cytogenet Genome Res 2002;97:171.

8. Mehenni H, Gehrig C, Nezu J, et al. Loss of LKB1 kinase activity in Peutz-Jeghers syndrome, and evidence for allelic and locus heterogeneity. Am J Hum Genet 1998;63:1641.

9. Olschwang S, Boisson C, Thomas G. Peutz-Jeghers families unlinked to STK11/LKB1 gene mutations are highly predisposed to primitive biliary adenocarcinoma. J Med Genet 2001,30:356.

10. Burt RW, Jass J. Hyperplastic polyposis. In: Hamilton SR, Aaltonen LA, editors. World Health Organisation classification of tumours pathology and genetics. Berlin: Springer-Verlag; 2000. p. 135.

11. Liaw D, Marsh DJ, Li J, et al. Germline mutations of the PTEN gene in Cowden disease, an inherited breast and thyroid cancer syndrome. Nat Genet 1997;16:64.

12. Marsh DJ, Dahia PL, Zheng Z, et al. Germline mutations in PTEN are present in Bannayan-Zonana syndrome. Nat Genet 1997;16:333.

13. Pilarski R. Cowden syndrome: a critical review of the clinical literature. J Genet Couns 2009;18:13.

14. Carlson GJ, Nivatvongs S, Snover DC. Colorectal polyps in Cowden's disease (multiple hamartoma syndrome). Am J Surg Pathol 1984;8:763.

15. Chen YM, Ott DJ, Wu WC, et al. Cowden's disease: a case report and literature review. Gastrointest Radiol 1987;12:325.

16. Marra G, Armelao F, Vecchio FM, et al. Cowden's disease with extensive gastro-intestinal polyposis. J Clin Gastroenterol 1994;18:42.

17. Nelen MR, Kremer H, Konings IB, et al. Novel PTEN mutations in patients with Cowden disease: absence of clear genotype-phenotype correlations. Eur J Hum Genet 1999;7:267.

18. Marsh DJ, Coulon V, Lunetta KL, et al. Mutation spectrum and genotype-pheno-type analyses in Cowden disease and Bannayan-Zonana syndrome, two hamar-toma syndromes with germline PTEN mutation. Hum Mol Genet 1998;7:507.

19. Tsou HC, Teng DH, Ping XL, et al. The role of MMAC1 mutations in early-onset breast cancer: causative in association with Cowden syndrome and excluded in BRCA1-negative cases. Am J Hum Genet 1997;61:1036.

20. Zhou XP, Waite KA, Pilarski R, et al. Germline PTEN promoter mutations and dele-tions in Cowden/Bannayan-Riley-Ruvalcaba syndrome result in aberrant PTEN protein and dysregulation of the phosphoinositol-3-kinase/Akt pathway. Am J Hum Genet 2003;73:404.

21. Chibon F, Primois C, Bressieux JM, et al. Contribution of PTEN large rearrange-ments in cowden disease: a multiplex amplifiable probe hybridisation (MAPH) screening approach. J Med Genet 2008;45:657.

22. Groden J, Thliveris A, Samowitz W, et al. Identification and characterization of the familial adenomatous polyposis coli gene. Cell 1991;66:589.

23. Nishisho I, Nakamura Y, Miyoshi Y, et al. Mutations of chromosome 5q21 genes in FAP and colorectal cancer patients. Science 1991;253:665.

24. Friedl W, Caspari R, Sengteller M, et al. Can APC mutation analysis contribute to therapeutic decisions in familial adenomatous polyposis? Experience from 680 FAP families. Gut 2001;48:515.

25. Powell SM, Petersen GM, Krush AJ, et al. Molecular diagnosis of familial adenomatous polyposis. N Engl J Med 1993;320:1982.
26. van der Luijt RB, Khan PM, Vasen HF, et al. Molecular analysis of the APC gene in 105 Dutch kindreds with familial adenomatous polyposis: 67 germline mutations identified by DGGE, PTT, and southern analysis. Hum Mutat 1997;9:7.
27. Aretz S, Stienen D, Uhlhaas S, et al. Large submicroscopic genomic APC deletions are a common cause of typical familial adenomatous polyposis. J Med Genet 2005;42:185.
28. Bunyan DJ, Eccles DM, Sillibourne J, et al. Dosage analysis of cancer predisposition genes by multiplex ligation-dependent probe amplification. Br J Cancer 2004;91:1155.
29. De Rosa M, Scarano MI, Panariello L, et al. Three submicroscopic deletions at the APC locus and their rapid detection by quantitative-PCR analysis. Eur J Hum Genet 1999;7:695.
30. Nielsen M, Bik E, Hes FJ, et al. Genotype-phenotype correlations in 19 Dutch cases with APC gene deletions and a literature review. Eur J Hum Genet 2007; 15:1034.
31. Sieber OM, Lamlum H, Crabtree MD, et al. Whole-gene APC deletions cause classical familial adenomatous polyposis, but not attenuated polyposis or "multiple" colorectal adenomas. Proc Natl Acad Sci U S A 2002;99:2954.
32. Poulsen ML, Bisgaard ML. MUTYH associated polyposis (MAP). Curr Genomics 2008;9:420.
33. Nielsen M, Hes FJ, Nagengast FM, et al. Germline mutations in APC and MUTYH are responsible for the majority of families with attenuated familial adenomatous polyposis. Clin Genet 2007;71:427.
34. Knudsen AL, Bisgaard ML, Bulow S, et al. Attenuated familial adenomatous polyposis (AFAP). A review of the literature. Fam Cancer 2003;2:43.
35. Al-Tassan N, Chmiel NH, Maynard J, et al. Inherited variants of MYH associated with somatic G:C-> T:A mutations in colorectal tumors. Nat Genet 2002;30:227.
36. Aretz S, Uhlhaas S, Goergens H, et al. MUTYH-associated polyposis: 70 of 71 patients with biallelic mutations present with an attenuated or atypical phenotype. Int J Cancer 2006;119:807.
37. Enholm S, Hienonen T, Suomalainen A, et al. Proportion and phenotype of MYH-associated colorectal neoplasia in a population-based series of Finnish colorectal cancer patients. Am J Pathol 2003;163:827.
38. Isidro G, Laranjeira F, Pires A, et al. Germline MUTYH (MYH) mutations in Portuguese individuals with multiple colorectal adenomas. Hum Mutat 2004;24:353.
39. Sieber OM, Lipton L, Crabtree M, et al. Multiple colorectal adenomas, classic adenomatous polyposis, and germ-line mutations in MYH. N Engl J Med 2003;348:791.
40. Wang L, Baudhuin LM, Boardman LA, et al. MYH mutations in patients with attenuated and classic polyposis and with young-onset colorectal cancer without polyps. Gastroenterology 2004;127:9.
41. Cheadle JP, Sampson JR. MUTYH-associated polyposis—from defect in base excision repair to clinical genetic testing. DNA Repair (Amst) 2007;6:274.
42. Eliason K, Hendrickson BC, Judkins T, et al. The potential for increased clinical sensitivity in genetic testing for polyposis colorectal cancer through the analysis of MYH mutations in North American patients. J Med Genet 2005;42:95.
43. Bouguen G, Manfredi S, Blayau M, et al. Colorectal adenomatous polyposis associated with MYH mutations: genotype and phenotype characteristics. Dis Colon Rectum 2007;50:1612.

44. Jaeger E, Webb E, Howarth K, et al. Common genetic variants at the CRAC1 (HMPS) locus on chromosome 15q13.3 influence colorectal cancer risk. Nat Genet 2008;40:26.

45. Jaeger EE, Woodford-Richens KL, Lockett M, et al. An ancestral Ashkenazi haplotype at the HMPS/CRAC1 locus on 15q13-q14 is associated with hereditary mixed polyposis syndrome. Am J Hum Genet 2003;72:1261.

46. Tomlinson I, Rahman N, Frayling I, et al. Inherited susceptibility to colorectal adenomas and carcinomas: evidence for a new predisposition gene on 15q14-q22. Gastroenterology 1999;116:789.

47. Cao X, Eu KW, Kumarasinghe MP, et al. Mapping of hereditary mixed polyposis syndrome (HMPS) to chromosome 10q23 by genomewide high-density single nucleotide polymorphism (SNP) scan and identification of BMPR1A loss of function. J Med Genet 2006;43:e13.

48. Hampel H, Frankel WL, Martin E, et al. Feasibility of screening for Lynch syndrome among patients with colorectal cancer. J Clin Oncol 2008;26:5783.

49. Hampel H, Frankel WL, Martin E, et al. Screening for the Lynch syndrome (hereditary nonpolyposis colorectal cancer). N Engl J Med 2005;352:1851.

50. Aaltonen LA, Peltomaki P, Leach FS, et al. Clues to the pathogenesis of familial colorectal cancer. Science 1993;260:812.

51. Aaltonen LA, Peltomaki P, Mecklin JP, et al. Replication errors in benign and malignant tumors from hereditary nonpolyposis colorectal cancer patients. Cancer Res 1994;54:1645.

52. Boland CR, Thibodeau SN, Hamilton SR, et al. A National Cancer Institute Workshop on Microsatellite Instability for cancer detection and familial predisposition: development of international criteria for the determination of microsatellite instability in colorectal cancer. Cancer Res 1998;58:5248.

53. Rodriguez-Bigas M, Boland C, Hamilton S, et al. National Cancer Institute Workshop on Hereditary Nonpolyposis Colorectal Cancer Syndrome: meeting highlights and Bethesda guidelines. J Natl Cancer Inst 1997;89:1758.

54. Muller W, Burgart LJ, Krause-Paulus R, et al. The reliability of immunohistochemistry as a prescreening method for the diagnosis of hereditary nonpolyposis colorectal cancer (HNPCC)—results of an international collaborative study. Fam Cancer 2001;1:87.

55. Thibodeau SN, French AJ, Roche PC, et al. Altered expression of hMSH2 and hMLH1 in tumors with microsatellite instability and genetic alterations in mismatch repair genes. Cancer Res 1996;56:4836.

56. Acharya S, Wilson T, Gradia S, et al. hMSH2 forms specific mispair-binding complexes with hMSH3 and hMSH6. Proc Natl Acad Sci U S A 1996;93:13629.

57. Fishel R. The selection for mismatch repair defects in hereditary nonpolyposis colorectal cancer: revising the mutator hypothesis. Cancer Res 2001;61:7369.

58. Jascur T, Boland CR. Structure and function of the components of the human DNA mismatch repair system. Int J Cancer 2006;119:2030.

59. Kadyrov FA, Dzantiev L, Constantin N, et al. Endonucleolytic function of MutLalpha in human mismatch repair. Cell 2006;126:297.

60. Harfe BD, Minesinger BK, Jinks-Robertson S. Discrete in vivo roles for the MutL homologs Mlh2p and Mlh3p in the removal of frameshift intermediates in budding yeast. Curr Biol 2000;10:145.

61. Vasen H, Mecklin J-P, Khan P, et al. The international collaborative group on hereditary non-polyposis colorectal cancer. Dis Colon Rectum 1991;34:424.

62. Vasen H, Watson P, Mecklin J-P, et al. New clinical criteria for hereditary nonpo lyposis colorectal cancer (HNPCC, Lynch syndrome) proposed by the International Collaborative Group on HNPCC. Gastroenterology 1999;116:1453.

63. Barnetson RA, Tenesa A, Farrington SM, et al. Identification and survival of carriers of mutations in DNA mismatch-repair genes in colon cancer. N Engl J Med 2006;354:2751.

64. Chen S, Wang W, Lee S, et al. Prediction of germline mutations and cancer risk in the Lynch syndrome. JAMA 2006;296:1479.

65. Balmana J, Stockwell DH, Steyerberg EW, et al. Prediction of MLH1 and MSH2 mutations in Lynch syndrome. JAMA 2006;296:1469.

66. Lynch HT, de la Chapelle A. Hereditary colorectal cancer. N Engl J Med 2003; 348:919.

67. Palomaki GE, McClain MR, Melillo S, et al. EGAPP supplementary evidence review: DNA testing strategies aimed at reducing morbidity and mortality from Lynch syndrome. Genet Med 2009;11:42.

68. Baudhuin LM, Burgart LJ, Leontovich O, et al. Use of microsatellite instability and immunohistochemistry testing for the identification of individuals at risk for Lynch syndrome. Fam Cancer 2005;4:255.

69. Boland CR, Koi M, Chang DK, et al. The biochemical basis of microsatellite instability and abnormal immunohistochemistry and clinical behavior in Lynch syndrome: from bench to bedside. Fam Cancer 2008;7:41.

70. Shia J. Immunohistochemistry versus microsatellite instability testing for screening colorectal cancer patients at risk for hereditary nonpolyposis colorectal cancer syndrome. Part I. The utility of immunohistochemistry. J Mol Diagn 2008; 10:293.

71. Hampel H, Frankel W, Panescu J, et al. Screening for Lynch syndrome (hereditary nonpolyposis colorectal cancer) among endometrial cancer patients. Cancer Res 2006;66:7810.

72. Senter L, Clendenning M, Sotamaa K, et al. The clinical phenotype of Lynch syndrome due to germ-line PMS2 mutations. Gastroenterology 2008;135:419.

73. Chao EC, Velasquez JL, Witherspoon MS, et al. Accurate classification of MLH1/MSH2 missense variants with multivariate analysis of protein polymorphisms-mismatch repair (MAPP-MMR). Hum Mutat 2008;29:852.

74. Lindor NM, Rabe K, Petersen GM, et al. Lower cancer incidence in Amsterdam-I criteria families without mismatch repair deficiency: familial colorectal cancer type X. JAMA 2005;293:1979.

75. Balaguer F, Castellvi-Bel S, Castells A, et al. Identification of MYH mutation carriers in colorectal cancer: a multicenter, case-control, population-based study. Clin Gastroenterol Hepatol 2007;5:379.

76. Lubbe SJ, Webb EL, Chandler IP, et al. Implications of familial colorectal cancer risk profiles and microsatellite instability status. J Clin Oncol 2009;27:2238.

77. Nielsen M, Joerink-van de Beld MC, Jones N, et al. Analysis of MUTYH genotypes and colorectal phenotypes in patients With MUTYH-associated polyposis. Gastroenterology 2009;136:471.

78. Severin MJ Genetic susceptibility for specific cancers. Medical liability of the clinician. Cancer 1999;86:2564.

Role of Surgery in Familial Adenomatous Polyposis and Hereditary Nonpolyposis Colorectal Cancer (Lynch Syndrome)

Kerrington D. Smith, MD[a], Miguel A. Rodriguez-Bigas, MD, FACS[b],*

KEYWORDS

- Colorectal cancer • Herditary colorectal cancer
- Prophylactic surgery • Familial adenomatous polyposis
- Lynch syndrome • HNPCC

Surgery remains the mainstay of treatment for patients who develop colorectal cancer (CRC) in the setting of a hereditary CRC syndrome. In patients with a hereditary CRC syndrome, surgery can be prophylactic, therapeutic with curative intent, and, in some cases, palliative. The type and extent of surgical resection in familial adenomatous polyposis (FAP) and in the Lynch syndrome is influenced by differences in the natural history of carcinogenesis between the two syndromes and by the effectiveness of and patient compliance with available surveillance strategies. In this article, the surgical options for the management of patients with FAP and Lynch syndrome are discussed.

FAMILIAL ADENOMATOUS POLYPOSIS

Adenomatous polyposis was first observed in the mid-eighteenth century, and by 1900 its familial association was recognized. In the 1980s, FAP was linked to deletion of chromosome 5q[1] in a region that mapped to the adenomatous polyposis coli (*APC*)

[a] Division of Surgical Oncology, Dartmouth-Hitchcock Medical Center, One Medical Center Drive Lebanon, NH 03756, USA
[b] Department of Surgical Oncology, Unit 444, University of Texas MD Anderson Cancer Center, 1515 Holcombe Boulevard, Houston, TX 77030, USA
* Corresponding author.
E-mail address: sdjackso@mdanderson.org (M.A. Rodriguez-Bigas).

Surg Oncol Clin N Am 18 (2009) 705–715
doi:10.1016/j.soc.2009.07.006
1055-3207/09/$ – see front matter. Published by Elsevier Inc.

surgonc.theclinics.com

gene.[2,3] Germline mutations in the *APC* gene are associated with the development of classic FAP, which is responsible for the clinical phenotype characterized by the development of severe polyposis at a young age. However, the phenotype of patients with FAP can vary from the classic patients with hundreds or thousands of colorectal adenomas to attenuated FAP (AFAP) with a paucity of adenomas (20–100). Not all patients with FAP will have a family history of the syndrome. Approximately 20% to 30% of these patients will present as the index cases in their families.[4] Most patients with no family history of FAP will present with symptoms such as rectal bleeding and diarrhea. Bulow[5] reported a 60% incidence of CRC in patients with symptomatic FAP. In the era of endoscopic surveillance, the median age at diagnosis of adenoma is approximately 16 years.[4,6] In untreated patients, the mean age of CRC diagnosis and CRC death have been reported to be 39 and 42 years, respectively.[7] In AFAP, CRC will generally occur in the early to mid-50s.

The phenotypic manifestations of FAP are not limited to the large bowel. There are extracolonic manifestations, such as desmoid tumors, fundic gland polyps, duodenal adenomas, and others.[6] There are fairly clear associations between the genotype and phenotype in FAP. Patients with *APC* mutations between codons 1250 and 1464 have been associated with profuse polyposis (>5000 polyps).[8] It is within this region of the *APC* gene that the most common mutation is found. This mutation is in codon 1309 and is associated with severe polyposis and early-age-onset CRC.[9,10] AFAP has been associated with mutations at the extreme ends of the *APC* gene, in exons 3,4,5, and 15 and in exon 9.[11–15]

Surgery for FAP

The surgical options for patients with FAP include abdominal colectomy and ileorectal anastomosis (IRA), restorative proctocolectomy and ileal J-pouch anal anastomosis (IPAA), and total proctocolectomy (TPC) and ileostomy. The latter procedure should be reserved for patients with rectal cancer whose sphincters cannot be preserved, for the rare patient in whom an ileal pouch will not reach to perform an ileoanal anastomosis, and for those patients with poor sphincter function. TPC will not be further discussed. Prophylactic surgery in FAP has been shown to be effective in improving survival.[16]

Factors that may influence the type of procedure to be performed include patient factors, disease factors, and physician (surgeon) factors (**Table 1**). Each of these factors needs to be considered in the decision-making process. Patient factors include age of the patient, psychological well-being, signs and symptoms, and patient preference. The diagnosis of FAP with colorectal adenomas does not mean the need to perform surgery immediately. The risk of having a carcinoma at an age less than 20 years is approximately 1%.[17] Therefore, in the case of an asymptomatic at-risk or mutation carrier patient who has been diagnosed with adenomas on surveillance, if that individual and his family understand that there is a small risk for cancer, then it is the practice of the authors to try to wait until the patient finishes at least his or her high school education

Table 1	
Factors to consider in the surgical decision in FAP	
Timing of the Surgery	**Type of Procedure**
• Signs and symptoms	• Number and location of polyps
• CRC risk	• CRC
• Education	• Molecular genetics
• Psychological well-being	• Desmoid tumors, female fecundity

before performing surgery. However, if the patient is symptomatic with diarrhea, failure to thrive, and/or bleeding, then surgery should not be postponed. Disease factors include extent of polyposis; presence or absence of cancer (including metastases); extracolonic manifestations; and, in some situations, genotype. Patients with severe polyposis or CRC will likely present with signs and symptoms. Even if there are no signs and symptoms, patients with severe polyposis should not have their surgical procedure postponed.

If the patient presents with metastatic disease from a colon cancer it may be advisable to perform a less complex procedure (IRA) that deals with the cancer so that treatment for metastatic disease can be addressed. If the metastatic disease is addressed and the patient does well, then if necessary, the rectum can be addressed at a later time and a J pouch can be constructed.

Total abdominal colectomy and IRA

Total abdominal colectomy with IRA consists of removal of the abdominal colon and a primary anastomosis to the rectum. The advantage of this procedure is that it is less complicated than an IPAA and generally there is better function than after an IPAA. The disadvantage of this procedure is that the rectum remains in situ. Therefore, there is a risk of cancer developing in the rectal stump. The risk for rectal cancer has been reported to be anywhere from 15% to 40%. This widespread range is a function of the length of rectum and/or sigmoid colon left at the time of colectomy; the length of follow-up of the patient; and, in part, poor patient selection for the procedure. It has been suggested that with better patient selection for an IRA most patients will keep their rectum. In the "prepouch era" there was no patient selection for prophylactic surgery because the only alternatives of treatment were TPC or IRA. Thus, poor candidates for IRA, such as patients with the rectum carpeted with polyps or patients with colon cancer, would undergo the procedure because it was the only alternative to avoid a permanent stoma. Bulow and colleagues[18] and Church and colleagues[19] have demonstrated that with better patient selection in the "pouch era" the risk of rectal cancer in patients undergoing IRA is less than 10%. Better endoscopic surveillance may also be a factor that has contributed to a lower rectal cancer risk in the "pouch era". An IRA does not preclude an IPAA in the future if needed. The experience of the surgeon is paramount in the success of surgery, especially in more complex procedures, such as IPAA.

When making the surgical decision, the phenotype of the patient is another factor to consider. It has been reported that the risk of proctectomy after an IRA is more than 50% in patients with greater than 20 rectal adenomas or greater than 1000 colonic adenomas at the time of the original surgery (**Table 2**).[19] The genotype of the patient has also been implicated in later proctectomy after IRA. Patients with *APC* mutation 3' of codon 1250 and those with mutations in codons 1309 and 1328 were at a higher

Table 2	
Risk of subsequent proctectomy after abdominal colectomy and IRA	
Number of Adenomas	**Risk of Proctectomy (%)**
<5 rectal and <1000 colon	0
5–20 rectal	13
>20 rectal	54

Data from Church J, Burke C, McGannon E, et al. Predicting polyposis severity by proctoscopy: how reliable is it? Dis Colon Rectum 2001;44(9):1249–54.

risk of losing their rectums in follow-up because of cancer.[20,21] Bertario and colleagues[9] reported a higher risk for rectal cancer in patients with mutations in codons 1250 to 1464. IRA is the procedure of choice in patients with AFAP because these patients will present with colonic polyps or cancer, mainly right-sided with relative rectal sparing.

Restorative proctocolectomy and Ileal pouch anal anastomosis (IPAA)

IPAA is considered by some as the procedure of choice for the treatment of FAP. It consists of removing the entire colon and rectum down to the levators and performing an IPAA. There are several factors to consider while performing an IPAA. These include the type of pouch (whether J or S pouch), whether to perform a mucosectomy, and whether to handsow or to staple the anastomosis. Even though most surgeons will perform a diverting ileostomy, it has been reported that this may not be necessary.

Restorative proctocolectomy with IPAA is technically more complex and may be associated with a worse functional outcome than a total colectomy with IRA.[22]

IPAA is performed in patients with profuse polyposis and in those with CRC where the sphincter is not involved. The pouch can be either a J pouch that is constructed with two 15- to 20-cm long limbs, which are then either stapled or handsewn to the anal canal, or an S pouch that is constructed with three 15-cm limbs and a 2-cm spout, which is handsewn to the anal canal. The advantage of the S pouch is that it will reach further into the anal canal than the J pouch. The main disadvantage is that if the spout is longer than 2 cm, there will be issues with evacuation of the pouch and the need to intubate to evacuate the pouch because of obstruction and kinking. In addition, the S pouch will take longer to construct.

Whether to perform a mucosectomy depends on surgeon preference and the presence of polyps in the anal canal. If there are polyps in the anal canal, it is preferable to perform a mucosectomy and a handsewn anastomosis. If there are no polyps, then the anastomosis can be stapled to the anal canal. Irrespective of the technique it is important to continue surveillance of the pouch, because cancers in the anal transitional zone have been reported, and the incidence of adenomas in the pouch can be as high as 75% at 15 years post-IPAA.[21,23] The incidence of neoplasia at the site of IPAA anastomosis has been reported to be 10% to 14% after mucosectomy and handsewn anastomosis and 28% to 31% after stapled anastomosis.[22] The complication rate and function after mucosal stripping and handsewn anastomosis is worse than that after stapled anastomosis.[24,25]

There have been reports suggesting that function after an IPAA is comparable to the function after an IRA. A meta-analysis of 12 studies that compared IRA with IPAA in patients with FAP has been published.[26] In this meta-analysis, functional outcomes, including bowel frequency and incontinence in 24 hours, nocturnal defecation, and nocturnal incontinence, favored IRA. Fecal urgency was experienced more frequently in patients undergoing IRA than in those undergoing IPAA.[26] There were no differences in dietary restriction or male sexual function. In terms of morbidity, there were no differences between the 2 procedures except for a higher reoperation rate within 30 days in patients who underwent IPAA.[26] Also there was a higher incidence of rectal cancer and loss of the rectum in patients who underwent an IRA.[26]

Other factors that may affect the choice of surgery include female fecundity. In a Scandinavian study it was reported that female fecundity decreased 46% in women undergoing IPAA for FAP, whereas there was no decrease in female fecundity in women with FAP undergoing IRA.[27] It has also been reported that desmoid tumors may pose a problem at the time of surgery for FAP and after an IRA. Patients with FAP are at risk for the development of desmoids, occurring in up to 9% to 29% of patients, and these desmoids are a major source of morbidity and mortality.[28,29] FAP-associated desmoids, in contrast to sporadic desmoids that are localized to the abdominal wall, commonly arise within the intra-abdominal mesentery.[30] Mesenteric involvement may preclude complete resection due to the morbidity of small bowel short gut or may preclude IPAA reconstruction due to mesenteric foreshortening. Therefore, patients undergoing an attempted restorative procedure should be informed of this possibility and the possibility of a permanent ileostomy.[19]

Occasionally, obesity may preclude adequate mobilization to perform an IPAA. In the Cleveland Clinic experience, obese patients who underwent IPAA had comparable pouch function to nonobese patients.[31] In that study, there was a higher risk of the development of wound infection and anastomotic separation, but there were less bowel obstructions in obese patients.

The minimally invasive approach to IRA and IPAA procedures is an attractive option for patients. Laparoscopic approaches may offer advantages, such as less pain, faster recovery time, and potentially a less traumatic procedure, which may lead to a decrease in desmoid tumor formation. A randomized trial that compared hand-assisted laparoscopic restorative proctocolectomy with conventional IPAA in patients with FAP and ulcerative colitis demonstrated similar functional outcomes and quality of life but longer operative times and increased cost in the former procedure.[32] A randomized controlled trial in Germany comparing laparoscopic and conventional IPAA in ulcerative colitis and FAP is accruing patients.[33]

Surveillance and Timing of Surgery

Surveillance based on genetic testing or annual flexible sigmoidoscopy of at-risk family members begins around puberty because the average age of onset of polyposis is 16 years. Patients with AFAP are recommended to undergo a full colonoscopy because of the predominance of right-sided polyposis.[1] There have been reports of effective chemopreventive agents in FAP, such as sulindac and celecoxib.[34,35] These agents should not be used as primary treatment for FAP. They should be used as adjuncts to surgery, as they do not prevent polyps from forming, but they decrease the size and number of polyps.

In summary, the timing and type of surgery for FAP must be individualized. Each individual and each situation is different. With the advent of molecular genetics, better patient selection, and advances in surgical techniques, patients with FAP have alternatives at the time of surgery, and these should be discussed with the patient. The treatment can be tailored to the situation and needs of the patient. It must be remembered that no matter what procedure is performed, these patients will need long-term surveillance not only of their rectum or pouch but also for other extracolonic manifestations.

HEREDITARY NONPOLYPOSIS COLORECTAL CANCER (LYNCH SYNDROME)

Hereditary nonpolyposis colorectal cancer (HNPCC) syndrome, also known as Lynch syndrome, is more common than FAP and accounts for approximately 2% to 3% of the total CRC burden.[36] Unlike FAP, tumors in patients with HNPCC mostly arise proximal to the splenic flexure, and not all patients with HNPCC will develop CRC. In mismatch repair mutation carriers, the lifetime risk of CRC has been reported to be 28% to 75% in men and 24% to 52% in women.[17] Endometrial cancer is the second most common cancer in Lynch syndrome. It has been reported to be the index cancer in women with Lynch syndrome in about 35% of the cases.[37] The lifetime risk of endometrial cancer ranges from 27% to 71%, which, in some studies, is higher than the risk of CRC.[17] Surgery in the Lynch syndrome as in FAP can be curative or palliative. As opposed to FAP, the role of prophylactic surgery in HNPCC is not clearly established, although it should be an option in selected situations.

Surgical Management of HNPCC

For surgical management, patients with Lynch syndrome can be divided into (1) those with newly diagnosed CRC, (2) those with a history of CRC treated with less than a total abdominal colectomy, (3) those at risk or who are mutation carriers who have yet to develop CRC, and (4) those with advanced disease (**Box 1**). As with FAP, minimally invasive surgery is gaining popularity in patients with HNPCC.

In women who have completed their families and/or are postmenopausal, hysterectomy and bilateral salpingo-oophorectomy should be considered.

Newly diagnosed colon or rectal cancer

Patients with HNPCC with newly diagnosed colon cancer may be treated with segmental colectomy or more extensive procedures with lifelong surveillance of the remaining bowel at an interval of every 1 to 2 years. Whether more extensive surgery, such as a total abdominal colectomy and IRA, or restorative proctocolectomy with IPAA (in rectal cancer where the sphincters can be saved), provides a survival benefit compared with less extensive resection is less clear. Because the risk of metachronous CRC is estimated to be 40% at 10 years and 72% at 40 years after resection of the primary CRC,[37–40] in general it is recommended to perform an abdominal colectomy and IRA at the time of initial surgery in patients with Lynch syndrome with newly diagnosed CRC. There are no data, either prospective or retrospective, that

---

Box 1
Surgical management of patients with HNPCC[a]

- Newly diagnosed colon cancer

  Segmental resection

  Abdominal colectomy and IRA

- Newly diagnosed rectal cancer

  Segmental resection

  Segmental resection (abdominoperineal resection or TPC and ileostomy)[b]

  Restorative proctocolectomy with IPAA

- History of CRC treated with segmental resection

  Surveillance

  Completion colectomy

  Chemoprevention studies if available

- Mutation carriers with no CRC

  Surveillance

  Prophylactic colectomy as an option

  Chemoprevention studies if available

In Females who have completed their families and/or are postmenopausal consider hysterectomy and bilateral salpingo-oophorectomy.
[a] Mutation carriers.
[b] If poor sphincter function and/or sphincters involved.

demonstrate an improvement in survival in patients undergoing a more extensive procedure rather than a segmental resection. A mathematical model that compares segmental resection with more extended resections has been reported.[41] In this model, life expectancy was improved in younger patients with early CRC undergoing extended resections compared with older patients with similar staged tumors or patients with lymph node involvement irrespective of age. An IRA does not eliminate the risk of cancer in the rectum, which has been reported to be from 3% to 12%.[42,43] Therefore, surveillance of the rectum should be performed every 1 to 2 years. The main drawback of an IRA is the increased frequency of bowel movements compared with a segmental colectomy. Over time, most patients will adapt. Segmental colectomy and IRA are straightforward procedures with low morbidity and mortality.

Rectal cancer represents the index cancer in 20% to 31% of patients with HNPCC.[44,45] In individuals with rectal cancer, segmental resections (such as low anterior resection and abdominoperineal resections) or more extensive procedures (such as IPAA or TPC and ileostomy) can be considered. Whether the sphincters can be preserved depends on the sphincter involvement. In addition, the functional status of the sphincter muscles and patient preferences should also be considered in the decision making. If at the time of diagnosis of rectal cancer it is determined that the patient will benefit from neoadjuvant therapy, then surgery should proceed after such therapy.

Previous segmental resection

The management of the patient with segmental colectomy who is diagnosed with HNPCC, can entail prophylactic completion colectomy, surveillance, or, if available, participation in chemoprevention trials. There are no data to suggest that completion colectomy will improve the survival in these patients. Therefore, most of these patients undergo annual or biennial colonoscopies.

Mutation carriers who have not as yet developed CRC

The role of prophylactic colectomy in Lynch syndrome is not established as it is in FAP. Two mathematical models have been reported that compare prophylactic colectomy with surveillance. In one model, a survival advantage of 12 and 24 months was reported if colectomy was performed at the age of 30 years.[46] In the other, if colectomy was performed at age 25 years, the survival benefit was 19.6 months.[47] There are specific situations in which prophylactic colectomy should be considered in HNPCC. Patients whose colon cannot be regularly examined because of tortuosity or poor patient compliance or those patients with disabling psychological symptoms secondary to the fear of developing cancer are some of the examples in whom prophylactic colectomy may play a role in HNPCC. However, patients must understand that cancer can develop in the remaining rectum and in other extracolonic sites associated with the syndrome.

Mutation carriers with adenomas

The adenoma to carcinoma sequence is accelerated in the Lynch syndrome.[48] In individuals with adenomas, treatment options include endoscopic polypectomy (if possible) with surveillance or surgical resection as discussed for those with newly diagnosed CRC. The size and number of adenomas, the frequency of recurrent or metachronous adenomas, the risk of interval cancers, and the morbidity of endoscopic polypectomy and prophylactic surgery are some of the factors to be considered in the decision making.

Individuals with metastatic disease

It is not uncommon to encounter a patient with the Lynch syndrome with metastatic disease. In this situation, the treatment should be defined as potentially curative versus palliative. If surgery is indicated, whether curative or palliative, in the absence of any data to support a survival advantage of performing more extensive resections than a segmental resection, the authors usually prefer a segmental resection and surveillance, if indicated, because of the lower morbidity compared with an IRA. The advantages and disadvantages of IRA and IPAA are similar to patients with FAP, except that desmoid tumors are not associated with HNPCC.

Patients with Microsatellite Instability in their Tumors

Microsatellite Instability (MSI-H) is the hallmark of CRC in the Lynch syndrome. In younger individuals, the presence or absence of MSI-H in their tumor may help in the choice of surgery. Approximately 30% of patients with CRC younger than 30 years will carry a germline mutation in *MLH1* or *MSH2*.[34,49] In these individuals, if the tumor is MSI-H, the chance of finding a mutation in either of these mismatch repair genes is approximately 60%.[34,49] In patients younger than 50 years with MSI-H tumors, the chance of carrying a mutation in *MLH1* or *MSH2* is about 30%.[34,50] Thus patients aged less than 50 years with MSI-H tumors should be considered for more extensive procedures at the time of the primary surgery. That is not the case for older individuals with MSI-H tumors, because the instability will most likely be caused by methylation of the *MLH1* promoter and thus will be considered as sporadic cancers.

Surgical Options for Women with HNPCC

Endometrial cancer has emerged as the second most common cancer associated with HNPCC. In women with HNPCC, the lifetime risk of endometrial cancer is 27% to 71%,[17,51] and in women harboring mutations in mismatch repair genes, the lifetime risk of ovarian cancer is 12%.[52] The median age for the diagnosis of these gynecologic malignancies is in the fifth to sixth decade of life.[53] Women with HNPCC with CRC may benefit from surgical removal of the uterus to prevent the development of endometrial cancer and the removal of the ovaries to prevent the development of ovarian cancer. A retrospective study that compared a cohort of women with germline mutations in mismatch repair genes who underwent prophylactic surgery with another cohort of patients under surveillance demonstrated a significant decrease in the risk of endometrial cancer and ovarian cancer in the group treated with prophylactic surgery. Endometrial cancer developed in 33% of the control group and 0% in women who underwent prophylactic hysterectomy, whereas 5% of women in the control arm developed ovarian cancer compared with 0% in the group treated with prophylactic surgery.[54] For women undergoing colorectal surgery, prophylactic total abdominal hysterectomy with bilateral salpingo-oophorectomy should be offered if childbearing is complete or if the patient is postmenopausal. Such patients should have the opportunity to be evaluated by a gynecologic oncologist to discuss prophylactic surgery. When an endometrial biopsy has not been performed preoperatively, the uterus should be opened and examined intraoperatively. The decision to perform surgical staging of endometrial or ovarian cancer with sampling of regional lymph nodes is based on the results of intraoperative frozen section.[24]

SUMMARY

Surgeons must recognize the importance of a detailed family cancer history in the workup of patients presenting with CRC. An appreciation of the natural history, genetics, and extracolonic manifestations of the 2 most common hereditary cancer syndromes will allow an informed discussion of the treatment options, including the risks and benefits for prophylactic surgery and the efficacy of lifetime surveillance for metachronous cancers. As minimally invasive techniques are advanced, previous impediments to risk-reducing surgery that surrounded the invasiveness of the procedure will be lessened. In the absence of prospective trials to determine the efficacy of surveillance and surgical strategies, such decisions must continue to be guided by international expert consensus guidelines. Surgical decisions ultimately must be individualized to accommodate clinical presentation and patient preferences.

REFERENCES

1. Herrera L, Kakati S, Gibas L, et al. Gardner syndrome in a man with an intestinal deletion of 5q. AM J Med Genet 1986;25(3):473–6.
2. Bodmer WF, Bailey CJ, Bodmer J, et al. Localization of gene for familial adenomatous polyposis on chromosome 5. Nature 1987;328(1613):614–6.
3. Leppert M, Dobbs M, Scambler P, et al. The gene for familial adenomatous polyposis maps to the long arm of chromosome 5. Science 1987;238(4832):1411–3.
4. Burt R, Neklason DW. Genetic testing for inherited colon cancer. Gastroenterology 2005;128(6):1696–716.
5. Bulow S. Results of national registration of familial adenomatous polyposis. Gut 2003;52(5):742–6.
6. Campbell WJ, Spence RA, Parks TG. Familial adenomatous polyposis. Br J Surg 1994;81(12):1722–33.
7. Bussey HJR. Familial polyposis coli. Baltimore: The Johns Hopkins University Press; 1975.
8. Nagase H, Miyoshi Y, Horii A, et al. Correlation between the location of germ-line mutations in the APC gene and the number of colorectal polyps in familial adenomatous polyposis patients. Cancer Res 1992;52(14):4055–7.
9. Bertario L, Russo A, Sala P, et al. Multiple approach to the exploration of genotype-phenotype correlations in familial adenomatous polyposis. J Clin Oncol 2003;21(9):1698–707.
10. Caspari R, Friedl W, Mandl M, et al. Familial adenomatous polyposis: mutation at codon 1309 and early onset of colon cancer. Lancet 1994;343(8898):629–32.
11. Brensinger JD, Laken SJ, Luce MC, et al. Variable phenotype of familial adenomatous polyposis in pedigrees with 3' mutation in the APC gene. Gut 1998;43(4):548–52.
12. Nieuwenhuis MH, Vasen HF. Correlations between mutation site in APC and phenotype of familial adenomatous polyposis (FAP): a review of the literature. Crit Rev Oncol Hematol 2007;61(2):153–61.
13. Soravia C, Berk T, Madlensky L, et al. Genotype-phenotype correlations in attenuated adenomatous polyposis coli. Am J Hum Genet 1998;62(6):1290–301.
14. Spirio L, Olschwang S, Groden J, et al. Alleles of the APC gene: an attenuated form of familial polyposis. Cell 1993;75(5):951–7.
15. van der Luijt RB, Vasen HF, Tops CM, et al. APC mutation in the alternatively spliced region of exon 9 associated with late onset familial adenomatous polyposis. Hum Genet 1995;96(6):705–10.
16. Nugent KP, Spigelman AD, Phillips RK. Life expectancy after colectomy and ileorectal anastomosis for familial adenomatous polyposis. Dis Colon Rectum 1993;36(11):1059–62.

17. Vasen HFA, Möeslein G, Alonso A, et al. Guidelines for the clinical management of familial adenomatous polyposis (FAP). GUT 2008;57(5):704–13.
18. Bulow S, Bulow C, Vasen H, et al. Colectomy and ileorectal anastomosis is still an option for selected patients with familial adenomatous polyposis. Dis Colon Rectum 2008;51(9):1318–23.
19. Church J, Burke C, McGannon E, et al. Risk of rectal cancer in patients after colectomy and ileorectal anastomosis for familial adenomatous polyposis: a function of available surgical options. Dis Colon Rectum 2003;46(9):1175–81.
20. Vasen HF, van der Luijt RB, Slors JF, et al. Molecular genetic tests as a guide to surgical management of familial adenomatous polyposis. Lancet 1996; 348(9025):433–5.
21. Wu JS, Paul P, McGannon EA, et al. APC genotype, polyp number, and surgical options in familial adenomatous polyposis. Ann Surg 1998;227(1):57–62.
22. Remzi FH, Church JM, Bast J, et al. Mucosectomy vs. stapled ileal pouch-anal anastomosis in patients with familial adenomatous polyposis: functional outcome and neoplasia control. Dis Colon Rectum 2001;44(11):1590–6.
23. Parc YR, Olschwang S, Desaint B, et al. Familial adenomatous polyposis: prevalence of adenomas in the ileal pouch after restorative proctocolectomy. Ann Surg 2001;233(3):360–4.
24. Guillem JG, Wood WC, Moley JF, et al. ASCO/SSO review of current role of risk-reducing surgery in common hereditary cancer syndromes. J Clin Oncol 2006; 24(28):4642–60.
25. Ziv Y, Fazio VW, Church JM, et al. Stapled ileal pouch anal anastomoses are safer than handsewn anastomoses in patients with ulcerative colitis. Am J Surg 1996; 171(3):320–3.
26. Aziz O, Athanasiou T, Fazio VW, et al. Meta-analysis of observational studies of ileorectal versus ileal pouch-anal anastomosis for familial adenomatous polyposis. Br J Surg 2006;93(4):407–17.
27. Olsen KO, Juul S, Bulow S, et al. Female fecundity before and after operation for familial adenomatous polyposis. Br J Surg 2003;90(2):227–31.
28. Rodriguez-Bigas MA, Mahoney MC, Karakousis CP, et al. Desmoid tumors in patients with familial adenomatous polyposis. Cancer 1994;74(4):1270–4.
29. Speake D, Evans DG, Lalloo F, et al. Desmoid tumours in patients with familial adenomatous polyposis and desmoid region adenomatous polyposis coli mutations. Br J Surg 2007;94(8):1009–13.
30. Penna C, Tiret E, Parc R, et al. Operation and abdominal desmoid tumors in familial adenomatous polyposis. Surg Gynecol Obstet 1993;177(3):263–8.
31. Kiran RP, Remzi FH, Fazio VW, et al. Complications and functional results after ileoanal pouch formation in obese patients. J Gastrointest Surg 2008;12(4): 668–74.
32. Maartense S, Dunker MS, Slors JF, et al. Hand-assisted laparoscopic versus open restorative proctocolectomy with ileal pouch anal anastomosis: a randomized trial. Ann Surg 2004;240(6):984–91 [discussion: 991–2].
33. Antolovic D, Kienle P, Knaebel HP, et al. Totally laparoscopic versus conventional ileoanal pouch procedure–design of a single-centre, expertise based randomised controlled trial to compare the laparoscopic and conventional surgical approach in patients undergoing primary elective restorative proctocolectomy–LapConPouch-Trial. BMC Surg 2006;6:13.
34. Giardiello FM, Brensinger JD, Petersen GM. AGA technical review on hereditary colorectal cancer and genetic testing. Gastroenterology 2001;121(1): 198–213.

35. Steinbach G, Lynch PM, Phillips RK, et al. The effect of celecoxib, a cyclooxygenase-2 inhibitor, in familial adenomatous polyposis. N Engl J Med 2000;342(26):1946–52.
36. Aaltonen LA, Salovaara R, Kristo P, et al. Incidence of hereditary nonpolyposis colorectal cancer and the feasibility of molecular screening for the disease. N Engl J Med 1998;338(21):1481–7.
37. Aarnio M, Sankila R, Pukkala E, et al. Cancer risk in mutation carriers of DNA-mismatch-repair genes. Int J Cancer 1999;81(2):214–8.
38. Jemal A, Siegel R, Ward E, et al. Cancer statistics, 2008. CA Cancer J Clin 2008; 58(2):71–96.
39. Lynch HT, de la Chapelle A. Hereditary colorectal cancer. N Engl J Med 2003; 348(10):919–32.
40. Watson P, Vasen HF, Mecklin JP, et al. The risk of extra-colonic, extra-endometrial cancer in the Lynch syndrome. Int J Cancer 2008;123(2):444–9.
41. de Vos tot Nederveen Cappel WH, Buskens E, van Duijvendijk P, et al. Decision analysis in the surgical treatment of colorectal cancer due to a mismatch repair gene defect. Gut 2003;52(12):1752–5.
42. de Vos tot Nederveen Cappel WH, Nagengast FM, Griffioen G, et al. Surveillance for hereditary nonpolyposis colorectal cancer: a long-term study on 114 families. Dis Colon Rectum 2002;45(12):1588–94.
43. Rodriguez-Bigas MA, Vasen HF, Pekka-Mecklin J, et al. Rectal cancer risk in hereditary nonpolyposis colorectal cancer after abdominal colectomy. International Collaborative Group on HNPCC. Ann Surg 1997;225(2):202–7.
44. Lee JS, Petrelli NJ, Rodriguez-Bigas MA. Rectal cancer in hereditary nonpolyposis colorectal cancer. Am J Surg 2001;181(3):207–10.
45. Möslein G, Nelson H, Thibodeau S, et al. Rectal carcinomas in HNPCC. Lagenbecks Arch Chir 1998;115:1467–9.
46. Vasen HF, Wijnen JT, Menko FH, et al. Cancer risk in families with hereditary nonpolyposis colorectal cancer diagnosed by mutation analysis. Gastroenterology 1996;110(4):1020–7.
47. Syngal S, Weeks JC, Schrag D, et al. Benefits of colonoscopic surveillance and prophylactic colectomy in patients with hereditary nonpolyposis colorectal cancer mutations. Ann Intern Med 1998;129(10):787–96.
48. Jass JR, Smyrk TC, Stewart SM, et al. Pathology of hereditary non-polyposis colorectal cancer. Anticancer Res 1994;14(4B):1631–4.
49. Farrington SM, Lin-Goerke J, Ling J, et al. Systematic analysis of hMSH2 and hMLH1 in young colon cancer patients and controls. Am J Hum Genet 1998; 63(3):749–59.
50. Lamberti C, Kruse R, Ruelfs C, et al. Microsatellite instability-a useful diagnostic tool to select patients at high risk for hereditary non-polyposis colorectal cancer: a study in different groups of patients with colorectal cancer. Gut 1999;44(6):839–43.
51. Lin KM, Shashidharan M, Thorson AG, et al. Cumulative incidence of colorectal and extracolonic cancers in MLH1 and MSH2 mutation carriers of hereditary nonpolyposis colorectal cancer. J Gastrointest Surg 1998;2(1):67–71.
52. Lu KH, Dinh M, Kohlmann W, et al. Gynecologic cancer as a "sentinel cancer" for women with hereditary nonpolyposis colorectal cancer syndrome. Obstet Gynecol 2005;105(3):569–74.
53. Rijcken FE, Mourits MJ, Kleibeuker JH, et al. Gynecologic screening in hereditary nonpolyposis colorectal cancer. Gynecol Oncol 2003;91(1):74–80.
54. Schmeler KM, Lynch HT, Chen LM, et al. Prophylactic surgery to reduce the risk of gynecologic cancers in the Lynch syndrome. N Engl J Med 2006;354(3): 261–9.

Index

Note: Page numbers of article titles are in **boldface** type.

A

B

C

Surg Oncol Clin N Am 18 (2009) 717–726
doi:10.1016/S1055-3207(09)00070-2
1055-3207/09/$ – see front matter © 2009 Elsevier Inc. All rights reserved.

surgonc.theclinics.com

Moving?

Make sure your subscription moves with you!

To notify us of your new address, find your **Clinics Account Number** (located on your mailing label above your name), and contact customer service at:

Email: journalscustomerservice-usa@elsevier.com

800-654-2452 (subscribers in the U.S. & Canada)
314-447-8871 (subscribers outside of the U.S. & Canada)

Fax number: 314-447-8029

Elsevier Health Sciences Division
Subscription Customer Service
3251 Riverport Lane
Maryland Heights, MO 63043

*To ensure uninterrupted delivery of your subscription,
please notify us at least 4 weeks in advance of move.

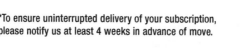

United States Postal Service

Statement of Ownership, Management, and Circulation
(All Periodicals Publications Except Requestor Publications)

1. Publication Title: Surgical Oncology Clinics of North America

2. Publication Number: 0 1 2 - 5 6 5

3. Filing Date: 9/15/09

4. Issue Frequency: Jan, Apr, Jul, Oct

5. Number of Issues Published Annually: 4

6. Annual Subscription Price: $218.00

7. Complete Mailing Address of Known Office of Publication (Not printer) (Street, city, county, state, and ZIP+4®)

Elsevier Inc.
360 Park Avenue South
New York, NY 10010-1710

Contact Person: Stephen Bushing

Telephone (Include area code): 215-239-3688

8. Complete Mailing Address of Headquarters or General Business Office of Publisher (Not printer)

Elsevier Inc., 360 Park Avenue South, New York, NY 10010-1710

9. Full Names and Complete Mailing Addresses of Publisher, Editor, and Managing Editor (Do not leave blank)

Publisher (Name and complete mailing address)

John Schrefer, Elsevier, Inc., 1600 John F. Kennedy Blvd. Suite 1800, Philadelphia, PA 19103-2899

Editor (Name and complete mailing address)

Catherine Bewick, Elsevier, Inc., 1600 John F. Kennedy Blvd. Suite 1800, Philadelphia, PA 19103-2899

Managing Editor (Name and complete mailing address)

Catherine Bewick, Elsevier, Inc., 1600 John F. Kennedy Blvd. Suite 1800, Philadelphia, PA 19103-2899

10. Owner (Do not leave blank. If the publication is owned by a corporation, give the name and address of the corporation immediately followed by the names and addresses of all stockholders owning or holding 1 percent or more of the total amount of stock. If not owned by a corporation, give the names and addresses of the individual owners. If owned by a partnership or other unincorporated firm, give its name and address as well as those of each individual owner. If the publication is published by a nonprofit organization, give its name and address.)

Full Name	Complete Mailing Address
Wholly owned subsidiary of	4520 East-West Highway
Reed/Elsevier, US holdings	Bethesda, MD 20814

11. Known Bondholders, Mortgagees, and Other Security Holders Owning or Holding 1 Percent or More of Total Amount of Bonds, Mortgages, or Other Securities. If none, check box. ☐ None

Full Name	Complete Mailing Address
N/A	

12. Tax Status (For completion by nonprofit organizations authorized to mail at nonprofit rates) (Check one)
The purpose, function, and nonprofit status of this organization and the exempt status for federal income tax purposes:
☐ Has Not Changed During Preceding 12 Months
☐ Has Changed During Preceding 12 Months (Publisher must submit explanation of change with this statement)

PS Form 3526, September 2007 (Page 1 of 3 (Instructions Page 3)) PSN 7530-01-000-9931 PRIVACY NOTICE: See our Privacy policy in www.usps.com

---

13. Publication Title: Surgical Oncology Clinics of North America

14. Issue Date for Circulation Data Below: July 2009

15. Extent and Nature of Circulation

			Average No. Copies Each Issue During Preceding 12 Months	No. Copies of Single Issue Published Nearest to Filing Date
a. Total Number of Copies (Net press run)			948	842
b. Paid Circulation (By Mail and Outside the Mail)	(1)	Mailed Outside-County Paid Subscriptions Stated on PS Form 3541. (Include paid distribution above nominal rate, advertiser's proof copies, and exchange copies)	333	326
	(2)	Mailed In-County Paid Subscriptions Stated on PS Form 3541 (Include paid distribution above nominal rate, advertiser's proof copies, and exchange copies)		
	(3)	Paid Distribution Outside the Mails Including Sales Through Dealers and Carriers, Street Vendors, Counter Sales, and Other Paid Distribution Outside USPS®	169	186
	(4)	Paid Distribution by Other Classes Mailed Through the USPS (e.g. First-Class Mail®)		
c. Total Paid Distribution (Sum of 15b (1), (2), (3), and (4))		▶	502	512
d. Free or Nominal Rate Distribution (By Mail and Outside the Mail)	(1)	Free or Nominal Rate Outside-County Copies Included on PS Form 3541	57	44
	(2)	Free or Nominal Rate In-County Copies Included on PS Form 3541		
	(3)	Free or Nominal Rate Copies Mailed at Other Classes Through the USPS (e.g. First-Class Mail)		
	(4)	Free or Nominal Rate Distribution Outside the Mail (Carriers or other means)		
e. Total Free or Nominal Rate Distribution (Sum of 15d (1), (2), (3) and (4))		▶	57	44
f. Total Distribution (Sum of 15c and 15e)		▶	559	556
g. Copies not Distributed (See instructions to publishers #4 (page #3))		▶	389	286
h. Total (Sum of 15f and g)		▶	948	842
i. Percent Paid (15c divided by 15f times 100)			89.80%	92.09%

16. Publication of Statement of Ownership

☐ If the publication is a general publication, publication of this statement is required. Will be printed in the October 2009 issue of this publication.   ☐ Publication not required

17. Signature and Title of Editor, Publisher, Business Manager, or Owner

Stephen R. Bushing   **Date** September 15, 2009

Stephen R. Bushing – Subscription Services Coordinator

I certify that all information furnished on this form is true and complete. I understand that anyone who furnishes false or misleading information on this form or who omits material or information requested on the form may be subject to criminal sanctions (including fines and imprisonment) and/or civil sanctions (including civil penalties).

PS Form 3526, September 2007 (Page 2 of 3)

Printed and bound by CPI Group (UK) Ltd, Croydon, CR0 4YY

03/10/2024

01040464-0013